LIVING CLAY

NATURE'S OWN MIRACLE CURE
CALCIUM BENTONITE CLAY

How To Treat and Cure 101 Ailments
Naturally with
Calcium Bentonite Clay

by Perry A~

Written by
Perry A~

Kyle, Texas 78640
www.LivingClayBook.com
1-866-883-1591

©2006 Perry A~

Printing History
First Printing – September, 2006
Second Printing – June, 2007
Third Printing – May, 2008
Fourth Printing – February, 2009

This book is manufactured in the United States of America
Print And Bind Direct!
Books@PrintAndBind.com

Cover Design by Cheryl McCoy

Library of Congress Card Catalog Number: Applied
Perry A~
Living Clay
ISBN: 1-887879-04-8

CONTENTS

FOREWORD

I was a skeptic at first – "Eat dirt?... You have got to be kidding!" That was my first response 12 short years ago when a friend offered me my first drink of Colloidal Clay. Today I eat, drink, bathe in, and apply topically, Living Clay. My experience has been the same as that of millions – to use it is to love it.

I am a layperson with no medical training. Although I do have a four-year degree, I feel blessed not to have been encumbered with a formal medical education. Had I been, I feel certain that somewhere along that 12 year trek some well-meaning, in-the-know soul would have instructed me that no good could come from eating clay. Fortunately for me, I spent the past 12 years eating clay and learned the truth.

The information in this book has been gathered from many sources. Much of it is my personal opinion and recommendations based on my own use. Much of the information has come from other clay users in the form of personal testimonials as well as historical accounts through the millennia. There is also a good deal of hard science from the leading researchers, both in the U.S. and around the world. With the recent surge of interest in Living Clay and all that it does, much more attention is now being directed towards the study of Living Clay.

This book is not intended to be used as a traditional medical reference work. If you are seeking medical advice – as defined by the FDA's criteria for 'medical advice' – please consult your medical physician. This book is about an all-natural curative mineral – Calcium Bentonite Clay – Living Clay. All referenced treatment protocols are those recommended and used by those who have used Living Clay as suggested. I invite you to make your own decisions about using this remarkable clay.

Now, enjoy the read and remember to take clay with you wherever you go.

The Author

INTRODUCTION

How many times have you seen a new ad on TV for the latest and greatest drug to hit the market only to learn that the "potential side effects" are worse than the problem you are trying to cure? I use to scoff at such warnings until I learned first hand all about the pesky "potential side effect" known as anal seepage...Suffice to say I would rather have kept my indigestion.

Today, there's rarely a day that goes by that we don't hear on the news or read in print of a new lawsuit against a major pharmaceutical company due to their miracle-cure drug somehow killing many people. Their stock response of, "...oh, but we told you one of the potential side effects could be your untimely death through heart attack or stroke. And you do know, of course, that our miracle-cure drug was studied and approved by the FDA, whose trials proved beyond a doubt that more people lived than died. But please know we understand your frustration..."

And then there was clay...Living Clay!

What if...just what if there was a natural substance to be found on our planet that really would fix what ails you and not harm what's not broken? And what if it fixed a multitude of ailments? What if it cured most anything wrong with your health? What if this miracle substance actually removed from your body all sorts of diseases, bacteria, fungi, parasites, chemicals, toxins and virals – yes, even viruses! But that's impossible, isn't it. It must be because the major pharmaceutical companies have told us it is impossible. Our entire medical industry then reinforces that belief and in turn we too know it can't be true...

But what if...just what if we all, as a society, had simply bought into the big lie?

And it's from this point of realization that we can again begin to seek the truth. Part of the hard reality of this truth is that for the last 70-80 years we've been hoodwinked about the efficacy of natural curatives.

This book is the result of my own awakening to one specific natural curative substance. Someone who I used to refer to as "my good friend, the Snake Oil Salesman" introduced me to it. Today I consider myself one of the leading advocates of this modern day, yet age old curative – Living Clay! Not just any clay, but more specifically Natural Calcium Bentonite Clay.

Since my awakening and conversion about 12 years ago, I have been on a personal crusade to inform others of the inherent miracles of this unique Living Clay.

Throughout this book you will learn about the miracle for yourself. I will remind you from time to time, that it is of utmost importance to use the clay yourself. I drink liquid clay or eat the hydrated clay daily. I apply hydrated clay to cuts, bruises, rashes and abrasions. I use clay as a cleanser in the shower, even "shampooing" my hair with it. I believe in clay.

You will learn the hard science behind Calcium Bentonite Clay and why it is effective for so many ailments. You will hear from physicians, MD's, OD's, scientists, laypeople, academics, children and even animals – well, at least the animals owners. There is no other substance on our planet that does what Living Clay can do. You will learn about the 6,000 years of documented history of clay cures. And I will offer some thoughts on what I believe someone's life will look like when using Living Clay extensively, from birth to death.

Is your quality of life dramatically improved with a lifetime of Living Clay use? Is ageless beauty actually possible without the knife and toxic chemicals? The answer to these questions and many more is a resounding YES!

First of all, Living Clay does not "cure" in a traditional sense. Clay is a catalyst that assists the body in detoxification and in removing positive charged ions from the body. In turn, Living

Clay creates a better platform for the body to begin healing itself. It propels the immune system to a healthy balance and strengthens the body to a higher point of resistance to all that attacks it. Secondly, it acts as a stimulus and as such increases circulation. Thirdly, it balances the body's pH. Living Clay is safe, gentle and pure. Natural Calcium Bentonite Clay has not been treated in any fashion.

Living Clay maintains its molecular integrity. It does not break down and assimilate into the body. It maintains a molecular whole as it passes through the body acting like a little vacuum cleaner, sucking up positive charged ions and carrying them out of the body. Since Living Clay is not digested and assimilated as it passes through the alimentary canal, the clay and the absorbed positive charged ions are both eliminated together. It also pulls toxins through the skin when applied topically and in clay baths. When used topically the clay, along with the positive charged ions removed through the skin, are washed off together. Clay baths are becoming more and accepted as a modality for detoxification due to their extreme effectiveness and their ability to detox and stimulate the lymphatic system, which acts as a filtering system for the body.

The study of Living Clay is fascinating. It is a 'living element' therefore capable of change through the millennia. This is also what makes clay so versatile and broad spectrum in it's various treatments of the body. Like a chameleon, clay adapts to its environment. It seems to know where to go and what to do, all without additional directions. The Native Americans say clay has a 'wisdom' of its own. I agree with this astounding observation after seeing so many remarkable and seemingly unexplainable results from taking and using Calcium Bentonite Clay.

As a result, in 1994 I began several years of study on Calcium Bentonite Clay. Frankly, I was surprised at the volume of material I found readily available on the subject. There were books, websites, videos, scientific papers, thousands of years of historical accounts, all singing the praises of this "newly discovered" miracle of Living Clay.

What I soon learned was that this specific clay has been a leading healing agent since time immemorial – at least until Bayer invented aspirin.

My hope is to assist in the return of Living Clay to the mainstream. In 1938 Raymond Dextreit first published *Our Earth, Our Cure*. Ran Knishinsky published *The Clay Cure* in 1998. During this 60-year span Calcium Bentonite Clay took a back seat to what became traditional, modern day medicine. Fortunately, over the past 10 years, natural medicine has experienced a dramatic resurgence. Our society has awakened from its drug-induced slumber and today realizes, with limited exception, we have been sold quite a bill of goods.

This book is a must read for anyone seeking a better quality of life…And that's the bottom line to all of this – use Living Clay and the quality of your life will improve. I'm referring to improved physical health, improved insight, improved mental acumen, and even a deeper sense of your own spiritual connection.

Now, go drink some clay!

LIVING CLAY AND HOW IT WORKS

I like keeping things simple...easy to understand. My intent is to reduce some relatively complicated scientific explanations into everyday language using analogies we can all understand.

I'll begin with the most basic fact of all – all clay is volcanic ash. When a volcano erupts and the lava flows down the side of the volcanic cone, the ash is blown high, oftentimes miles, high into the sky. Slowly it settles to the ground, sometimes nearby, sometimes hundreds of miles away, and in extreme cases it can circumvent the globe.

Volcanic ash—clay—falls into seven separate and distinct family groups. Within these seven families there are thousands of different types of mineral compositions, each unique and serving vastly different purposes in our world.

Kaolin clays are best known for their uses in anti-diarrheal products such as Kaopectate. While it absorbs toxins and bacteria to a limited extent, as do most clays, Kaolin clay acts primarily as a bulking agent. Some health food companies of late have begun selling Kaolin as a mineral supplement. I do not recommend natural Kaolin for any purpose other than severe diarrhea.

Illite clays are known for their commercial applications. It is a dirty green mineral clay found in marine settings. Some cosmeceutical companies use this industrial clay in their "mud" formulations due to it's high content of long dormant microbials and other sea life residue. Illite is generally a non-swelling clay. Pure finds of Illite are rare. Illites break down into the metal and mineral elements and is absorbed into the body. I would never recommend illities for internal ingestion.

Chlorite clays are known for their abrasive and cleansing properties. Cleaner and scrubbing powders are typical products made from this clay. Never use this caustic, abrasive clay on your body.

Vermiculite clays are used for making china, pottery and other like applications such as porcelain finishes on metals. While Vermiculite is not recommended for use on the body, there is one company selling a USP grade Vermiculite for internal use. This is not an adsorbent, swelling clay, and has both a positive and negative charge. Therefore I do not recommend it.

Mixed group clays occur when a volcano spews ash from several different internal plate formations. It is not uncommon to find mixed group clay formation at many mines or quarries.

Lath-formed clays are yet another mixed form and a typical use is fired bricks for construction. It is not suitable for use on the body.

Smectite clays compromise 99% of all clays used for health purposes today. Smectites are unique in that they swell while absorbing and adsorbing positive charged ions. It is the favored clay for health and dietary use as well as for many industrial applications.

Smectites are more complicated clays and have a higher exchange capacity than the other six family groups of clay. It has the unique ability to adsorb and absorb toxins at a greater rate than any other group. Calcium Bentonite Clay is a member of the Smectite family.

The term "Bentonite" is ambiguous. As defined by geologists, it is a rock formed of highly colloidal and pliable clays composed mainly of Montmorillonite, a clay mineral of the Smectite group, and is produced by *in situ* devitrification of volcanic ash (Parker, 1988.) The transformation of ash into Bentonite apparently takes place only in water (certainly seawater, probably alkaline lakes, and possibly other fresh water) during or after deposition (Grim, 1969; Patterson & Murray, 1983).

By extension, the term Bentonite is often incorrectly applied commercially to any pliable, colloidal and swelling clay regardless of its geological origin. Such clays are ordinarily composed largely of minerals of the Montmorillonite group but are not necessarily true Bentonite clays.

The term "Montmorillonite" is also ambiguous and is used both for a group of related clay minerals and for a specific member of that group (Bates & Jackson, 1987). In this case, Smectite is more appropriate.

ABSORPTION VS. ADSORPTION

The two words look alike but their difference is critical in understanding the functions of clay minerals.

Adsorption is the process by which substances stick to the outside surface of a clay molecule similar to the way a strip of Velcro works.

Absorption is the process of drawing substances into the clays internal molecular structure – similar to a sponge absorbing water.

The process by which substances are absorbed or adsorbed is through their electrical ionic charge. If you remember when you were young and you played with horseshoe magnets, when you placed like poles together – negative-to-negative and positive-to-positive – the two magnets repelled. When you placed opposite poles together – negative to positive – they actually pulled toward each other and stuck together.

The ionic charge of pure, natural Calcium Bentonite Clay is negative. This unique clay adsorbs and absorbs positive charged ions in a similar fashion. Most everything that attacks our bodies – bacteria, virals, fungi, diseases, toxic chemicals, etc. – is of a positive ionic charge. The beauty of Living Clay is that it is blind. It doesn't know an eczema molecule from a staph bacteria molecule, or a viral molecule. What it does know is a positive charge. As we apply hydrated Calcium Bentonite Clay topically to our bodies or drink liquid Calcium Bentonite Clay, its only function is to draw to itself positive charged molecules, which it holds like a magnet, both internally and externally, until we wash them from our bodies or pass them through our bodies. Calcium Bentonite Clay literally removes positive charged molecules that attack our bodies from our bodies.

ALL CLAYS ARE NOT CREATED EQUAL

Within the Smectite family there are hundreds of different types of clays, each consisting of between 8 and 145 minerals. As mentioned earlier, the most common sub family is Montmorillonite. Further along the Montmorillonite family tree are the various Bentonites. It's from the Smectite family tree that we find the broadest spectrum healing modality on our planet – Calcium Bentonite Clay.

Montmorillonite Clay was named after the town of Montmorillon in France where it was first identified. Its common name is French Green and you will see it packaged under several different brands today and available in many health food stores. Green swelling clays are known for their remarkable healing properties. Not to say that non-swelling clays are not good also, but due to the molecular makeup the swelling clays have a greater drawing or detoxing potential.

According to Raymond Dextreit, an expert on clays and author of the book, *Our Earth, Our Cure*, the green family of clays is the most desirable and the most preferable type recommended for ingestion.

Bentonite Clay was named after the town of Ft. Benton, Wyoming where it was first identified by a miner named John Pascal. His product was branded as Pascalite, which is a form of non-swelling calcium based Bentonite Clay.

Calcium Bentonite Clay is the most rare form of clay in the Smectite family. There have been only a few finds throughout the history of mines, which contained pure, natural, Calcium Bentonite Clay. Even though Sodium Bentonite, and Calcium

Bentonite Clay are cousins from the same family genesis, they are as different as night and day in efficacy and intended uses.

There are ten things you should ask of any clay you are considering for topical or internal use for health purposes.

Is it a Calcium based Bentonite?

Is the clay milled to at least a 325-screen mesh particle?

Is the pH at least 9.5?

Is it a Living Clay capable of adsorbing and absorbing positive charged ions?

Is it a green swelling clay of the Montmorillonite/Smectite group?

Is it tasteless and odorless?

Is its efficacy, its ionic ratio at least 20 to 1? (Drawing power)

Is it an all-natural, clean clay, direct from the mine source which has not been processed or purified in any fashion?

Is it a clay from a mine protected from the elements?

Is it a clay that expands and absorbs to a 1 to 3 ratio in volume? One part dry clay to three parts water.

WHY ARE THESE TEN QUESTIONS IMPORTANT?

It is critical that when you ingest clay it be Calcium based as opposed to Sodium based. Demand from any clay company that you be given a copy of the MSDS sheet and a copy of the Mass Gas Spectrometer Test results. These two documents will give you the specific mineral composition of their clay. Any company who refuses to give you this data is hiding something from you.

Most Sodium Bentonite is suitable for commercial and industrial uses such as sealing farm ponds, sealing asphalt and in oil rig mud pits.

A good quality Calcium Bentonite Clay should contain the following as its top three minerals.

Silica Oxide

Calcium Oxide

Magnesium Oxide

In addition it should contain no more than 2.5% in sodium. One popular Sodium Bentonite contains 9% sodium! When doing a cleanse, detox or tackling any health related issue, the last thing you want to do is to ingest substantial amounts of salt.

It is also important that the clay be pure, clean and natural direct from the source mine—preferably a subsurface mine that has been protected from the natural elements. Most clays that claim to be 100% pure have been cleaned using either a heat process or a hydration process to "wash" out impurities. Both processes can take a 95% pure clay to a "100%" pure state, but in doing so reduces the efficacy from around 15 to 1 down to 5 to 1. In their attempt to make a purity claim they are actually destroying the natural healing properties. Read labels carefully for any notation of the clay having been cleaned, processed, filtered, recharged or tampered with in any fashion other than milling.

Clays are all milled to various degree of "fineness." This fineness number typically runs from 50 to 325-screen mesh. A 50-screen mesh feels like fine grain sand while a 325 mesh is almost as fine as talcum powder. The finer the mesh the better the milling process and in turn the better it hydrates when water is added. Suspension as a colloidal is cleaner, quicker and more highly charged. If taken internally in a capsule form it is imperative that Calcium Bentonite Clay be screened to at least a 325 mesh so that it assimilates into a colloidal in the shortest time possible after ingestion. I recommend you not buy any Calcium Bentonite Clay that is milled to larger than a 325-screen mesh.

The pH of your Calcium Bentonite Clay is crucial. One of its greatest blessings to your health is its ability to increase your pH from acid to alkaline. While all clays are alkaline, only 2-3 are 9.3 to 9.7 in their natural state. I recommend you select a Calcium Bentonite Clay with the highest pH available.

Naturally you want tasteless, odorless clay that is creamy smooth when hydrated. Unprotected clays tend to pick up odors. Be wary of clays with strong odors.

Lastly, and of paramount importance, is a clay's efficacy rate – how well it works. This piece of information is provided in a ratio from such as 10 to 1. This means the following: a clay with a 10 to 1 efficacy rating removes 10 times it's molecular weight in positive charged ions from your body. By contrast, a clay with a 3 to 1 efficacy rating would remove 3 times its molecular weight in positive charged ions (the bad stuff that attacks our bodies). In this example a 10 to 1 ratio when compared to a 3 to 1 ratio means the first clay would be over 3 times as effective as the second.

Clays capable of exchanging ions are called Living Clays or Active Clays. Clays' ability to absorb and adsorb directly affect their efficacy rate. Green swelling clays from the Montmorillonite/Smectite group are known as healing clays because of this trait.

There are three clays on the market today with an efficacy ratio greater than 12 to 1. Few natural Calcium Bentonite Clays have a 31 to 1 ratio. I recommend you read the literature carefully and call the company reps to find the best products among the many second best on the market today. If they don't know the efficacy rate and mineral content, I would consider it a doubtful source. Remember, the purpose of clay when used on a daily basis is to continually remove positive charged ions – the things that attack our bodies. The very best clay to accomplish this goal is a pure natural Calcium Bentonite Clay with a pH of 9.0-9.7, a screen mesh of 325 and an efficacy ratio of at least 30 to 1.

That being said, knowing what clay to use, becomes the paramount question. I've looked at two clays, and swore by looking at them they were the same... And yet, the swelling properties were quite different, as were the tastes. They even look the same under a 10,000x microscope, as the screen mesh and minerals are the same, only in slightly different percentages.

Today there are many other technologies available for testing various clays. Most are very expensive. Kinesiology is a widely accepted practice and a BodyTalk System Practitioner can test your body's response to several different clays. For verifying results of metal contamination I recommend Hair Analysis and the Melisa Test, a blood test for metal sensitivity. The Melisa Test measures your immune system's (lymphocyte) activation when exposed to specific heavy metals.

NOW FOR A LITTLE MORE SCIENCE

The molecular shape of a Sodium Bentonite molecule is pyramidal in shape. Its molecular weight is the same as that of a Calcium Bentonite molecule. The difference is that a Calcium Bentonite molecule is shaped like a credit card – a large, very flat rectangle. Both have a negative ionic charge and both will absorb (soak up like a sponge) the same amount of positive charged ions. The difference is in the surface area where adsorption occurs (sticks to the surface like Velcro). The surface area of a Calcium Bentonite Clay molecule is 20 times that of a Sodium Bentonite Clay molecule, therefore the efficacy is greatly enhanced based on its adsorption rates.

Remember, the magic of Calcium Bentonite Clay lies in the fact it is a strongly negative charged ionic molecule. It "works" by drawing to itself positive charged ions, holding them within itself and on itself until the Calcium Bentonite Clay is washed from your body or passed through your body…I really do like keeping things simple…

For those desiring a more scientific explanation however, try this: You will hear clay referred to as a colloid. The dictionary defines colloid (k l'oid) [Gr.,=gluelike], a mixture in which one substance is divided into minute particles (called colloidal particles) and dispersed throughout a second substance. A pertinent example is mixing dry powder clay with water. For practical purposes I refer to it as hydrated clay. A swelling clay with water added at a 1 part clay to 3 parts water ratio is about the consistency of thick sour cream, depending on the amount of water added.

Colloidal particles are larger than molecules but too small to be observed directly with a traditional microscope; however, their shape and size can be determined by electron microscopy. In a true solution, the particles of dissolved substance are of molecular size and are thus smaller than colloidal particles; in a coarse mixture (e.g., a suspension) the particles are much larger than colloidal particles. Although there are no precise boundaries of size between the particles in mixtures, colloids, or solutions, colloidal particles are usually on the order of 10^{-7} to 10^{-5} cm in size.

The Scottish chemist Thomas Graham discovered (1860) that certain substances (e.g., glue, gelatin, or starch) could be separated from certain other substances (e.g., sugar or salt) by dialysis. He gave the name *colloid* to substances that do not diffuse through a semi-permeable membrane (e.g., parchment or cellophane). **Semi-permeable membrane** - A membrane that permits the passage of a solvent, such as water, but prevents the passage of the dissolved substance, or solute – the clay.

One property of colloid systems that distinguishes them from true solutions is that colloidal particles scatter light. The British physicist John Tyndall first explained the scattering of light by colloids, known as the Tyndall effect. When an ultramicroscope is used to examine a colloid, the colloidal particles appear as tiny points of light in constant motion; this motion, called Brownian movement, helps keep the particles in suspension. Absorption is another characteristic of colloids, since the finely divided colloidal particles have a large surface area exposed.

The particles of a colloid selectively absorb ions and acquire an electric charge. All of the particles of a given colloid take on the same charge (either positive or negative) and thus are repelled by one another. If an electric potential is applied to a colloid, the charged colloidal particles move toward the oppositely charged electrode; this migration is called electrophoresis. If the charge on the particles is neutralized, they may precipitate out of the suspension.

The above passages are for those who need a scientific explanation of how clay works and why it is not digested or absorbed into the bloodstream. This is what is meant when clay is referred to as maintaining its integrity. Thus, a colloid may be precipitated by adding another colloid with oppositely charged particles; the particles are attracted to one another, coagulate, and precipitate out. When clay is taken internally, because of its large surface area and negative charge, it dominates positive charged particles (toxins and bacteria) drawing them to it and carrying them out of the body.

Many people are concerned about natural metals in some clays. Any metals in Living Clays are never in isolated form and are not adsorbed into the body. Therefore the metals in a clays make up are not harmful, as the body does not digest them. This is why clay is known first and foremost as a strong, safe detoxifier. For clays with a high pH it is also known as a balancer bringing the body to a balanced state. Most people are naturally on the acidic side and acidity is the breeding ground for bacteria and diseases.

THE ENERGY OF CLAY

The following are excerpts from two excellent books on natural healing and Living Clay.

"If we go back to our base physical components, we can safely say that we are built from multitudes of particles held together by electrical bonds. Electrical forces are what hold atoms and molecules together. Chemical bonds and reactions depend on these electrical forces. Therefore, all chemical reactions are, in essence, reorganizations of electrical forces, which continue to be vital at body levels, i.e., tissues and organs. When this is all taken into account, a living organism is shown to be an extremely delicate and intricate electrical system." (Homeopathy for Everyone, 1987, Gibson & Gibson.)

"During illness, the vital force is weak and incapable of supporting the body and its functions. In health, however, the opposite occurs: the force is strong and is able to counteract sickness and decay. What keeps the immune system running is the energy that feeds it, the substance of life. The body will not run well, or will at least run with all sorts of mechanical problems, when there is no energy to support it.

When Living Clay is consumed, its vital force is released into the physical body and mingles with the vital energy of the body, creating a stronger, more powerful energy in the host. Its particles are agents of stimulation and transformation capable of withholding and releasing energy at impulse. The natural magnetic action transmits a remarkable power to the organism and helps to rebuild vital potential through the liberation of latent energy. When it is in contact with the body, its very nature compels it to release its vital force from which so many plants and animals feed.

Therefore, in order to create health, the body must be stimulated and restimulated by another working energy like Living Clay. When the immune system does not function at its best, the clay stimulates the body's inner resources to awaken the stagnant energy. It supplies the body with the available magnetism to run well.

Does this mean you have to be sick to take clay? No, not at all. The best-known characteristic of clay is that it "acts as needed." Living clay is said to propel the immune system to find a new healthy balance. Reactions are not forced, but rather triggered into effect, as they are needed. To put it in other words, clay strengthens the body to a point of higher resistance. In this way, the body's natural immune system has an improved chance of restoring and maintaining health." (The Clay Cure, 1998, Ran Knishinsky)

6,000 YEARS OF DOCUMENTED HISTORY OF LIVING CLAY

When I first began research on Living clay in earnest in 1994, I was pleasantly surprised to find a greater lineage of documented history on clay than virtually any other mineral. That being the case, I asked myself the question: If clay had been the single most used healing modality for countless centuries, how had it suddenly fallen from the map into obscurity? The answer was quite surprising…

What I found was that it really hadn't fallen off the map at all. In fact, what had happened in a well-orchestrated fashion, is that the major pharmaceutical companies had been buying Calcium Bentonite mining claims over the past 100 years, taking the mineral off the market. Then they began adding Calcium Bentonite Clay to their pharmaceuticals – not under the name of Calcium Bentonite Clay – but rather listing silica, calcium, magnesium, etc., as minerals in its medicine. In short, the pharmaceutical companies hijacked the finest natural curative in the world, changed its name, and put it in hundreds of their chemical concoctions.

Today, the active ingredient in most all stomach, gas, and acid remedies is Calcium Bentonite Clay. It is in Pepto Bismol, Tums, and Rolaids. It is in virtually every toothpaste on the market. Most recently it has been listed as an "inert binder" in pills of all kinds. The pharmaceutical companies may refer to it as an inert mineral binding agent, but the truth be known, it's what makes their chemical curatives actually work.

These companies know the powers of Living Clay and they have to a great degree been successful in securing the available resources and then using it to make their products work. What

I want you to know is that it is the gift of the Living Clay that is curing our bodies, the same as it has throughout history.

I've accumulated literally hundreds of references to the miracle of Clay during the past 10 years. I'm including many in this book. Taken as a body of historical reference they paint a very clear picture.

Fortunately, our society has begun a process of returning to natural remedies, having awakened from the industry induced slumber. Please allow these historical accounts and quotes to take root and to enrich your personal awakening, then consider picking 1 or 2 favorites and sharing them with your awakening friends.

In recently discovered medical texts inscribed in cuneiform, the first system of writing, researchers JoAnn Scurlock and Burton Anderson found that physicians of ancient Mesopotamia delivered surprisingly sophisticated health care using clay as their principal curative agent. Between 3500 – 150 A.D., physician/priests treated over 300 documented ailments with natural desert clay in the same fashion as is recommended today. The clay cuneiform text tablets state that methods of treatment included liquid clay and pill ingestion, rectal and vaginal suppositories, enemas, saturated ear tampons, transdermal patches, and salves spread on bandages. They were careful to keep surgical wounds clean with cotton bandages saturated with liquid clay.

Native Americans call it "Ee-Wah-Kee," meaning "Mud that Heals." Calcium Bentonite Clay has been used by indigenous cultures since before recorded history. The Amargosians (predecessors to the Aztecs), the Aborigines, and natives of Mexico and South America all recognized the healing benefits of clay.

Among the most famous clay-eaters in the animal kingdom are the parrots of the Amazon. In a recent National Geographic photo essay, it showed Scarlet Macaws, Blue and Gold Macaws, and hosts of smaller birds perched together by the hundreds eating clay along a riverbank. The parrots regular diet of clay allows them to eat toxic berries as a substantial portion of their diet. The clay detoxifies the berries as they are eaten and sets up an essential buffer in the parrots' bodies to protect them from being poisoned.

According to Jewish theology, the "Golem" was an eyeless, mouthless monster of a clay man who they raised to protect them from the "Goyem" who robbed and ransacked their villages.

"In the beginning God gave to every people a cup of clay, and from this cup they drank their life." - Native American Proverb.

The Hunza people drink extremely small amounts of glacial clay daily in their water supply, from birth to death, and it was not so long ago that these people were considered the healthiest people on Earth; the average 70 year old would be able to run circles around our Western 20 year olds.

The Pomo Indians of California consume Bentonite Clay with traditionally bitter and toxic types of acorns. The clay absorbs the toxins and eliminates the bitterness. These Indians are able to survive on the acorns as a food staple because of the clay.

Mahatma Gandhi imported thousands of tons of French Green Clay to India to cure intestinal ailments and overcome constipation.

In Fiji, one of the native tribes uses this cure for cholera: Leaves of an herb are placed in a jar of water with a ball of clay suspended above the preparation. The leaves are boiled; the ball of clay is crushed and stirred into the water. This mix is given to the patient to drink, and reportedly the cure rate is 100%.

In Guatemala, home of the St. Esquipulas shrine, 5.7 million "Holy" clay tablets are produced annually! The evolution of the shrine here may have "Christianized" clay eating. The tablets are seen as an extension of the power of the shrine. Upon eating the Holy clay tablets, cures of many illnesses have been reported, including ailments of the stomach, eyes, heart and pelvis. Interestingly, the Roman Catholic Church has indeed blessed medicinal clay tablets since the earliest days of Christianity, a millennium and a half before the statue of Saint Esquipulas was carved.

In Malaysia, women who want to bear children eat clay to help secure pregnancy.

In New Guinea, pregnant women eat clay because they believe it is good for fetal development.

In Russia, pregnant women place clay on their tongue to expedite birth and to facilitate easier expulsion of the after-birth. It is also used to combat morning sickness.

"Everything in Nature contains all the powers of Nature. Everything is made of one hidden stuff – Clay." - Ralph Waldo Emerson.

Clay is recognized worldwide as a treatment for diarrhea. In China, clay has been used for centuries as a cure for summer diarrhea and cholera. In 1712, Father Deutrecolle, a Jesuit missionary traveling through China, described the clay works there and mentioned that clay was used in treating diarrhea. In fact, as late as 1919, clay provided an invaluable medicine in the cholera epidemic that swept through China.

Long before recorded history, humans have used healing clays both internally and externally to cure illness, sustain life and promote general health. Ancient tribes of the high Andes, central Africa and the Aborigines of Australia used clay as a dietary staple, a supplement and as a curative for healing purposes.

In the second century A.D., Galen, the famous philosopher and physician, was the first to record the use of clay by sick or injured animals. He later recorded numerous cases of internal and external clay use in his book on Clay Therapy.

In ancient Arabia, Avicena, the "Prince of Doctors," taught hundreds of his students about the curative powers of Clay Therapy.

The Greek physician, Dioscorides, who was considered the engineer of medicine for the Roman Empire, attributed "God-like Intelligence" to the properties exhibited by clay used for therapeutic purposes.

The Essenes, keepers of the Dead Sea Scrolls, used clay for natural healing of a wide variety of illnesses and injuries. In fact, the caves Qumran where the scrolls were kept were Calcium Bentonite caves. The clay caves are today credited for their preservation.

The many benefits of clay were recognized by the Amargosians (who preceded the Aztecs) and the natives of Mexico and South America.

Various North American Indian tribes use clay for food, body purification, healing, in ceremonial events and as a form of currency to barter with other tribes.

Early French cultures used clay for nutrition and medicinal purposes. They touted the clay's healing effect on gum diseases, ulcers, rashes, dysentery, hemorrhoids, infected wounds and bites.

The 19th century German naturopath, Sebastian Kneipp, and fellow naturalist Adolph Just, accorded clay therapy a prominent position in their arsenal of Holistic Medicine due to the tremendous results they achieved using it.

Early in the 20th century, Julius Stump, a renowned German physician, successfully used clay therapy to cure Asiatic cholera. A contemporary, Dr. Meyer Camberg, used green clay to neutralize arsenic poisoning.

During WWI, German physicians offered clay therapy as a solution to food poisoning, dysentery, diarrhea and battle wound infection that was rampant among troops on both sides, greatly reducing mortality rates.

Russian scientists used clay to protect their bodies from radiation when working with nuclear material. Because it absorbs radiation so well, Bentonite Clay was chosen to dump into the Chernobyl reactors after the meltdown there.

The Egyptians used it to purify bodies for mummification. It was used extensively in Egypt on both the living and the dead.

In Switzerland and Germany, doctors made use of clay for healing purposes. In Davos, an important center for treatment of tuberculosis, patients were usually treated with clay; the whole thorax was daubed with a paste of very hot clay and this pack was kept on overnight. This treatment was credited with miraculous healings.

In the 16th century, the small village of Chatel-Guyen, France, became famous for its healing waters. Every day, at certain hours prescribed by a local doctor, people would go to various springs depending on their condition. Along with bathing in the waters and drinking prescribed amounts of the water, they would be treated to an "earth" bath, which consisted of freshly dug Living Clay which was heated so that when applied it would almost burn the skin. After 2-3 weeks of treatments, people left cured of a wide range of ailments including dysentery, gastro-intestinal troubles and removal of amoeba and parasites.

The earliest recorded find of a pure, natural Calcium Bentonite Clay was at the western side of the Dead Sea in Israel. Traces of Calcium Bentonite Clay remain today which enable scientists to validate its prior existence in substantial amounts, as do the caves at Qumran. Biblical references to "edible white stones" and eating of the hidden "manna" I believe refer to white Calcium Bentonite Clay in it's natural stone state and "manna" being a liquid colloidal form of Calcium Bentonite Clay mixed with honey for internal ingestion.

For 40 years, the Israelites consumed the white manna in order to spiritually prepare themselves for entry into Canaan, the Promised Land. Below are several biblical references to Clay, edible white stones and manna.

Exodus 16:15 "And when the children of Israel saw it, they said to one another, 'It is Manna': for they knew what it was.

And Moses said unto them, "This is the bread which the LORD hath given you to eat."

Exodus 16:31 "And the house of Israel called the name thereof Manna: and it was like coriander seed, white; and the taste of it was like wafers made with honey."

Exodus 16:33 "And Moses said unto Aaron, Take an urn, and fill it with an omer of Manna therein, and lay it up before the LORD, to be kept for your generations."

Exodus 16:34 "As the LORD commanded Moses, so Aaron laid it up before the testimony to be kept."

Exodus 16:35 "And the children of Israel did eat manna for 40 years, until they came to the land inhabited; they did eat manna, until they came to the borders of the land of Canaan."

Exodus 32:20 "And he took the Golden Calf which they had made and burnt it with fire, and ground it to a powder and strewed it upon the water, and made the children of Israel drink it."

Could the gold calf have been made from Monatomic Gold, which came from calcium Bentonite Clay? It would all fit!

We also know from Biblical history that Moses was the adopted son of a royal Egyptian family. Is it possible that the Divine Bread, or Manna, had its roots in ancient Egyptian alchemy?

Ancient Egyptian texts state that when the Pharaohs spiritually prepared themselves to enter the "Abode of the Immortals" (the Egyptian "Promised Land") they were fed clay. The sacred white substance was prepared in the "House of Life" by the Egyptian high priests and was considered "Food of the Gods."

The spiritual power of the clay is clearly indicated in the Egyptian texts. The Book of the Dead states, "Let there be given unto him clay and ale which have been issued in the Presence of Osiris, and he will forever be like the "Followers of Horus" (considered divine sage-priests).

The ancient Vedic tradition in India also sang the praises of a sacred white powder substance which, when mixed with water and honey, was called Soma, the nectar of immortality. Today, one of the world's largest deposits of White Bentonite Clay is being mined in the region where this verse was written.

Rig Veda 8:48 "I have tasted, as one who knows its secret, the honeyed (Soma) drink that inspires and grants freedom, the drink that all, both Gods and mortals, seek to obtain, calling it nectar. We have drunk the Soma, we have become immortal; we have gone to the light; we have found the Gods...These glorious drops are my health and salvation; they strengthen my joints as thongs do my cart. May these drops guard my foot lest it stumble and chase from my body all manner of ills. Well known Soma, stretch out our life spans so that we may live long. Enter within us for our well-being...Our weariness and pains are now far removed. Soma has surged within us mightily. The drops that we have drunk have entered our hearts turning immortal inside mortals. We have reached our goal. Life is prolonged!"

The collection, crushing, and milling of Soma are abundantly described in the Rig Veda. The chalklike stones would be collected by the dwellers of the region and brought to the alchemist – priests. The Soma would be crushed into pea-sized pieces; then ground with large stones into a fine powder. Several stages of grinding, washing, cooking and filtering are described. A woolen fleece was used as the final filter.

After crushing, grinding, washing and filtering, the Soma would be cooked in water. As the Soma began to "mature," it was said to become clothed in robes of milk. In other words, it assumed a white appearance, resembling milk or the moon. Due to its white color, it was often referred to in the Rig Veda as the "Milk of Heaven" or "Milk of God."

It is interesting to note that when monatomic elements are hydrated in water they quickly form a perfect colloidal that looks exactly like pure white milk.

Coming back close to home and moving to current times, one of the most fascinating natural formations on our planet is the Calcium Bentonite Clay Mountains near Shoshone, California. These mountains lie on the Western Shoshone Indian Reservation land. Over the past 1300, years medicine men from the Western Shoshone nation have carved out multi-room cave dwellings directly into the Calcium Bentonite Clay Mountains. These are sacred grounds and miraculous healings occur in these clay dwellings. The current Chief and Medicine Man of the Western Shoshone Nation, Chief Corbin Rainey, lives at his tribal compound about 8 miles south in Tecopa Springs, California. Chief Rainey uses Living clay extensively in his healings, both at his sacred healing center and in the caves themselves. The clay is considered sacred and Chief Rainey says its powers will remove any disease from the body and double a life span if ingested daily.

Finally, from the most read book in the World, the Bible, man was created from clay and Jesus healed the blind with clay.

John 9:6 When He had said these things, He spat on the ground and made clay with the saliva; and He anointed the eyes of the blind man with the clay.

John 9:7 And He said to him, "Go, wash in the pool of Siloam." So he went and washed, and came back seeing.

John 9:8 Therefore the neighbors and those who previously had seen that he was blind said, "Is not this he who sat and begged?"

John 9:9 Some said, "This is he," others said, "He is like him." He said, "I am he."

John 9:10 Therefore they said to him, "How were your eyes opened?"

John 9:11 He answered and said, "A man called Jesus made clay and anointed my eyes and said to me, 'Go to the pool of Siloam and wash.' So I went and washed, and I received sight."

John 9:12 Then they said to him, "Where is he?" He said, "I do not know."

John 9:13 They brought him who formerly was blind to the Pharisees.

John 9:14 Now it was Sabbath when Jesus made the clay and opened his eyes.

John 9:15 Then the Pharisees also asked him again how he had received his sight. He said to them, "He put clay on my eyes, and I washed, and I see."

And I personally believe there is a real simple explanation for the 600-900 year life spans spoken of extensively in the Old Testament, Calcium Bentonite Clay from the Dead Sea.

HOW TO TREAT AND CURE 101 AILMENTS NATURALLY

Clay and water...those two lifelines are all you will often need to return your body to a state of optimal health. This chapter will give you information on how to treat and cure over 101 ailments.

While we will focus on treatment modalities using only Calcium Bentonite Clay and water, many of you use clay in conjunction with other natural treatments such as herbs, nutrients, cleanses, or diets, all of which can be quite effective in their own right. None of the above can hurt the effectiveness of the clay, nor can any enhance the power of the clay. They can and do work in very different fashions and can, for the most part, work together without harm. That being said, it is my opinion that clay is most effective when used as a stand-alone .

For some of the ailments listed below, only a brief treatment protocol will be listed. For others, I have chosen to offer some of the whys and hows of Calcium Bentonite Clay's effectiveness to better explain the function of the clay in relation to the specific ailment and the body itself.

There are five primary treatment modalities with clay. Once you understand the different methods of applying Calcium Bentonite Clay, locate your ailment from the following alphabetical references beginning on page 28 and follow the simple basic directions.

The five types of treatments are as follows:

DRY POWDER APPLICATION

The dry powder Calcium Bentonite Clay application is the most basic. Simply apply dry powder by hand in the amount indicated by the treatment modality.

POULTICE (CLAY PACK)

To make a poultice – clay pack – mix the dry powder Clay into a heavy paste. Use approximately 1 part clay to 1 – 1 ½ parts water. Stir thoroughly with a wooden or plastic spoon (do not use metal). Allow to sit for several hours until the water is completely assimilated with the clay. Spread a thick layer of the clay paste onto a piece of cloth or gauze. Apply to the affected area. Repeat as indicated.

HYDRATED TOPICAL APPLICATION

To mix the dry powder of a swelling clay into a hydrated state, mix 1 part clay with 3 parts water depending on the clay you are using. A good swelling clay usually has a 1 to 3 ratio. Allow to stand a minimum of 12 hours. Mix thoroughly until a creamy consistency, similar to sour cream. This can be applied topically by hand to any part of the body, from a facial to a full body wrap.

24

LIQUID DRINK

To mix the liquid ingestible form of the clay, mix 1 part clay to 8 parts water. Use a juice bottle or sports bottle. Shake vigorously for 3-5 minutes, or until the clay remains suspended in the water. Let stand for about 1 hour and again shake vigorously for a second time. Shake again before each use.

Another alternative used by many is to stir, with a plastic or wooden spoon, 1 heaping teaspoon to 1 tablespoon of dry powder clay into an 8 oz. glass of water and drink it.

CLAY BATH

A clay bath can be prepared in 2 fashions. Pour 32-64 ounces (a quart to a half gallon) of prepared liquid clay directly into hot running bath water and stir by hand. Secondly, if using dry powder clay, turn the tap full open and hand cast 1-2 cups or more depending on what you want to accomplish, of the clay under the water tap. Stir by hand for a minute or so. Continue until dissolved or get in the tub and continue stirring as the tub fills, until fully dissolved.

We have found that there are three primary questions about Calcium Bentonite Clay use for healing purposes. The first has to do with warnings regarding use of clay, particularly when someone is taking physician prescribed medication. The second has to do with taking clay over extended periods of time, or as a life practice. And the third question concerns the possibility of dealing with a healing crisis. Please read the following carefully:

CLAY USE AND MEDICATION WARNING

If you are under a physician's care for a chronic ailment, taking life-supporting pharmaceutical medications, or medications containing metals, please consult with your physician prior to using clay. The clay can pull the metals from your body and reduce the efficacy of these life supporting pharmaceutical medications.

TAKING CLAY OVER TIME

Clay works best when taken over a long period of time. That's because its actions are subtle. Like a snowball rolling down the hill, it starts off small and slow. As it continues to roll, it soon picks up momentum and goes faster. Clay does not offer instant cures for all ailments, but history shows it can encourage the body to put up a better fight when taken over a long period of time.

When clay is taken for indefinite periods of time, it has no addictive qualities. This is a big concern for many who begin eating the clay. The effects can be so positive that it scares them into thinking they might need it forever. However, one can quit eating clay at any time. There are no withdrawal symptoms, and you will never need to enter a withdrawal program. Many people ask if clay is something they have to take for the rest of their life. The answer to the question, of course, is they don't have to; there is no risk in discontinuing its use. But, why not take something that is good and will help clean out your body? Especially in today's highly polluted world, the liver and kidneys are so overworked they never have a chance to rest. Taking a spoonful of Calcium Bentonite Clay every day helps keep the mind and body functioning in tip-top condition. To remain healthy, eat clay daily.

Ran Knishinsky suggests that the regular intake of liquid clay (typically one to three tablespoons daily, in divided doses) can produce other benefits including parasite removal from the intestines, allergy and hay fever relief, and elimination of anemia and acne. For example it reduces discomfort from allergies by quickly neutralizing allergens that would otherwise produce allergic reactions; and it reduces heartburn and indigestion by absorbing excess stomach acids.

In 'The Clay Cure,' Knishinsky writes that clay is part of his diet and he never skips a day without eating clay. He writes,

"When the immune system does not function at its best, the clay stimulates the body's inner resources to awaken the stagnant energy. It supplies the body with the available magnetism to run well. Clay is said to propel the immune system to find a new healthy balance and strengthens the body to a point of higher resistance."

HEALING CRISIS

As part of the healing process, the body will begin to discard toxic residues which have built up in the body over the years. During the initial phase of healing, as your body begins to clean house (detoxify) and your vital energy begins to repair and rebuild internal organs, you may experience a healing crisis.

You may feel worse before you feel better. As you continue to improve, you may begin a process called retracing. For example, if you used to get skin rashes, the rashes may reappear or get worse for a period of time as your body eliminates toxins through the skin. You may also experience an initial increase in urination, or you may feel more nervous. In actuality, you are not getting worse, you are actually getting better. Soon, usually in 1-3 days, you will reach a plateau of better health.

For example, a varicose ulcer will at first enlarge itself as the dead flesh of the periphery will fall off the surface, and pus or blood can appear. Pain may even increase for some time but it will decrease later and finally disappear with a definite closing of the ulcer and rebuilding of healthy tissues. We must not be afraid of these reactions; on the contrary, they are desirable, for they are a sign that the organism is responding to this intervention.

Sometimes an obstacle arises in clay treatment which can hinder its continuation; the appearance of red patches or eruptions accompanied by unbearable itching. The explanation is that perhaps acid substances flowing from internal regions pass through the tissues attracted by clay. The fact that this itching stops after clay applications are discontinued would confirm this hypothesis.

During the healing crisis, it is important to not suppress these temporary symptoms with drugs because they may interrupt the process. Do, however, use common sense and listen to your body.

One of the beauties of Calcium Bentonite Clay treatments is that is it not an exacting science. Simply get the clay in you and on you in any fashion you so choose. Remember, you can't use the clay wrong!

The protocols listed below are only recommendations. Feel free to use clay in any fashion that best suits your own personal needs or preferences.

For ailment listing please see the alphabetical index which can be found at the back of the book.

Now, go play in some clay and heal thyself!

ABRASIONS

For minor abrasions—scratches, cuts, nicks, general all round boo-boos—treat topically as follows. If the abrasion is bleeding, sprinkle some dry powder Calcium Bentonite Clay directly onto the bleeding area. This will speed the clotting process and protect the wound from infection. After bleeding has stopped, apply a thin layer of hydrated clay to the affected area and the area surrounding the abrasion. Pain should subside in minutes and healing time will be cut in half. Two to three times a day, the abrasion should be rinsed with water and a new application of clay applied. If warranted, the clay-covered abrasion may be covered with a band-aid or telfa pad.

ABSCESS – see Toothache

ACID REFLUX

Calcium Bentonite Clay diminishes acid reflux so quickly in some cases that many consider it nothing short of a miracle. One user who had suffered with acid reflux for over 30 years says that within 3 days of his first dose of liquid Calcium Bentonite Clay he has not suffered since from what had been his lifetime of discomfort!

Acid reflux is easily treated with daily ingestion of liquid Calcium Bentonite Clay.

For the first 3 days, drink 3 ounces of liquid Calcium Bentonite Clay in the morning and again just before lying down for bed. You may also drink an additional ounce just before and after any meals which cause you discomfort.

For the next 3 days, drink 1-2 ounces of liquid Calcium Bentonite Clay in the morning and again just before lying down for bed.

From this point forward, simply maintain the evening 1-2 ounce dose as needed to permanently remove acid reflux from your life.

ACIDIC SYSTEM – see pH Balance

ACNE

To effectively deal with any problem, you must first understand and eliminate the root cause of the problem. Acne is a sebaceous (below the surface of the skin) problem and therefore must be attacked from the inside out as well as topically. We must also understand exactly what causes acne in the first place.

WHAT CAUSES ACNE?

Oil glands are located deep in the skin. They are known as sebaceous glands.

Each oil gland is connected to a tiny canal that contains a hair. The base of this hair is called the follicle. Oil glands are also connected to open skin pores, which do not contain a follicle.

These glands produce oil (also known as sebum) that flows to the surface of the skin through these canals to lubricate the hair follicles and the surrounding skin. The openings of these canals are the skin pores.

Oily skin occurs when an overactive oil gland enlarges and overproduces oil. Acne develops when some of the pores (through which oil normally flows from the oil gland to reach the skin surface) become blocked, resulting in trapping of oil within the skin pores. Skin cells that have been shed from the lining of the skin pore bunch together and block the pores. A blackhead or whitehead will develop from this skin pore blockage.

WHAT CAUSES THE SEBACEOUS GLANDS TO OVERPRODUCE, RESULTING IN ACNE?

According to Randall Neustaedter, OMD, the androgenic hormones, particularly testosterone that increase at puberty, and the surge of premenstrual hormones, trigger increased production of sebum. The pores become clogged with both sebum and dead skin cells creating a prime breeding ground for bacteria. These bacteria and the breakdown products of sebum cause irritation and inflammation in the pores. The result is acne – blackheads, whiteheads, pustules, and cysts in the skin.

Karen Jessett, author of *Clear Skin*, says that food is also a factor. She states there is recent research pointing the finger at diet – eating refined carbohydrates and sugar leads to a surge in insulin and an insulin-like growth factor called IGF-1. This in turn leads to an excess of male hormones, which encourage the skin to excrete large amounts of sebum. This grease-like substance encourages the growth of bacteria responsible for acne.

Then there's the issue of hygiene. Generally speaking, acne is not caused by poor hygiene. Exceptions to this statement would be people such as auto mechanics who are often in contact with skin damaging toxins. But for most people, the problem is not poor hygiene. In fact, vigorous scrubbing of the face does more harm than good. It can actually stimulate the sebaceous glands to overproduce, thus exacerbating the problem!

Ran Knishinsky, author of *The Clay Cure*, recommends using clay internally as well as externally. The following is an excerpt from his book:

"The condition of the skin is a good indication of what is happening inside the body. Most people are not aware that the skin is the largest organ and a means of eliminating waste; each day waste passes through the pores of the skin. Everything that affects the body in turn affects the skin. When the body is full of toxic wastes and cannot eliminate them properly, various skin ailments may result. The only effective way to get rid of these conditions is by cleaning the body inside and out.

The clay enriches and cleanses the blood, prompting better circulation and allowing the skin to get rid of waste."

It's essential to battle the acne at its source, which is INSIDE the body. Dr. James Meschine, DC, writes:

"To understand the relationship between detoxification, intestinal cleansing and prevention of acne, we must first understand the relationship between our skin, the digestive system and excretory system.

AUTOINTOXICATION (also know as autotoxicosis, enterotoxication, intestinal intoxication, intestinal toxemia or self-poisoning) which means the toxins released by the decay process, brought on by bacteria, pass into the blood stream and travel to all parts of the body. Every cell in the body can be affected and many forms of sickness can result from it, including acne and other skin eruptions. Detoxification is a normal body process of eliminating or neutralizing toxins through the colon, liver, kidneys, lungs, lymph and skin."

Acne is surprisingly easy to clear up using Calcium Bentonite Clay internally and topically. The clay enriches and cleanses the blood, promoting better circulation and allowing the skin to get rid of the waste. Used as a topical treatment and a mask, it deep cleanses the skin, unclogging the pores and allowing the gland oil to flow freely and do its job.

My 21-year-old son, who had battled acne for about 5 years, completely cleared up his problem in one short week. The first 2-3 days he said he didn't think it was doing much for his skin. I heard from him 10 days later when he called me frantically asking that I send him another jar of "dirt." He said by day 7 of his internal and topical use, his acne had disappeared completely. Then he ran out of the clay and over the past couple of days, his pimples had started to return.

Take internally 2 ounces of the prepared liquid clay in the morning and at bedtime for the first 7 days. After that, drink 1 ounce daily in the morning as a life practice.

Treat the affected areas topically by using the hydrated clay as a thin film mask, twice daily for 3 days, morning and evening, then once daily for 3 additional days. Then once weekly as a life practice.

You may also treat those severe blemishes and postulates topically by applying "spot" treatments. Just dab some hydrated clay onto any persistent or infected acne blemishes and "wear" all day. Calcium Bentonite Clay can be worn as a thin cover up as well for bad blemishes. It masks as it cleans and purifies.

A thin facial mask may also be left on overnight at anytime. Simply rehydrate and wash off in the morning.

One national supplier of natural Calcium Bentonite Clay offers an amazing 3-week guarantee. If an acne sufferer uses their products, the liquid Calcium Bentonite Clay for internal cleanse and the hydrated Calcium Bentonite Clay for topical use, they guarantee even the worst case of acne to be cured in 3 weeks. Reportedly, they have never had a request for a refund. They also encourage their customers to buy the economical bulk powder and learn to mix their own liquid and hydrated clay. For less than the cost of a doctors visit and a round of acne prescription medications, you can now stop acne naturally – guaranteed! However, as noted earlier and due to FDA restrictions these curative claims cannot be made directly by the sellers of clay. They do, however, unconditionally guarantee your complete satisfaction with their products.

AGE SPOTS – see Lipofuscin Abnormalities

AGENT ORANGE DETOXIFICATION – see Detoxification, Full Body

AIDS – ACQUIRED IMMUNO DEFICIENCY SYNDROME (HIV)

AIDS is a virus! According to traditional medical beliefs – there are no cures for a virus…any virus…When using traditional treatment modalities such as pharmaceutical medications, this happens to be the case. They haven't yet figured out how to "kill" a virus and not kill the rest of your body. That's a big problem with traditional medicines – the carry over "kill factor."

All viruses consist of positive charged ions. They are aberrant, sick, often rapidly reproducing cells, which can quickly overcome healthy cells and organs. As you know, Calcium Bentonite Clay is a negatively charged ion. Clay's only function is to absorb and adsorb positive charged ions. Clay helps remove virals, including AIDS/HIV, from your body.

As with all major, life threatening ailments, we encourage you to consult with your doctor before altering any treatment program you are now on. Your condition may be so advanced, your body so ill, so dependant on your current treatment regimen, that you may do further harm by altering your current treatment. That being said…

Any viral can be removed from your body. In the case of AIDS, which is systemic, blood borne and all pervasive, we recommend the strongest, most aggressive approach possible – and the one, which is completely safe and can do no harm.

The 3-pronged attack with Calcium Bentonite Clay includes full body immersion baths, full body wraps and ingestion of the liquid clay. Throughout this treatment we ask you to monitor T-cell counts and viral antibody counts weekly so you can see your results and improvement.

Treatment regimen days 1-7

Morning – Drink 6 ounces liquid Calcium Bentonite Clay. Take a hot clay bath for 20 minutes.

Afternoon – Drink 6 ounces liquid Calcium Bentonite Clay. Do a full body Calcium Bentonite Clay wrap – head to toe. Leave on for 45-60 minutes. Shower off.

Evening – Drink 6 ounces liquid Calcium Bentonite Clay. Take a hot clay bath for 20 minutes.

Treatment regimen days 8-21

Morning – Drink 4 ounces liquid Calcium Bentonite Clay. Take a hot clay bath for 20 minutes.

Afternoon – Drink 4 ounces liquid Calcium Bentonite Clay. Do a full body Calcium Bentonite Clay wrap – head to toe. Leave on for 45-60 minutes. Shower off.

Evening – Drink 4 ounces liquid Calcium Bentonite Clay. Take a hot clay bath for 20 minutes.

Treatment Regimen days 22-45

Morning – Drink 2 ounces liquid Calcium Bentonite Clay

Afternoon – Drink 2 ounces liquid Calcium Bentonite Clay. Do a full body Calcium Bentonite Clay wrap – head to toe. Leave on for 45-60 minutes. Shower off.

Evening – Drink 2 ounces liquid Calcium Bentonite Clay. Take a hot clay bath for 20 minutes.

Treatment regimen days 46-90 may be modified depending on speed of recovery. Continue this regimen until all traces of AIDS virus have been removed.

Morning – 1 ounce liquid Calcium Bentonite Clay

Afternoon – 1 ounce liquid Calcium Bentonite Clay. Every second day do a full body Calcium Bentonite Clay wrap head to toe. Leave on for 45-60 minutes. Shower off.

Evening – 1 ounce liquid Calcium Bentonite Clay. Take a hot clay bath for 20 minutes.

Keep in mind with AIDS/HIV, clay works by actually drawing to itself, through its negative ionic charge, the positive charged AIDS viral molecule. It is absorbed into or adsorbed onto the clay molecule and held. It is then either passed through your body, or washed off of your body. And literally, down the drain it goes.

Monitor your progress, watch your T-cell counts begin to grow and expect a healthy life in a few short months. And remember, it's only a virus…

ALCOHOLISM

Alcoholism takes a toll on the entire body – both physically and emotionally. It is a disease, which essentially harms every major organ in our body. Calcium Bentonite Clay's benefit when tackling a body racked by alcoholism is first in its function of cleansing and detoxing the entire body, and secondly in setting the stage for the body to begin the healing process.

We recommend the following use of Calcium Bentonite Clay when setting aside alcohol.

Days 1-2

Morning – Drink 6-8 ounces liquid Calcium Bentonite Clay. Take a hot clay bath for 20 minutes. Apply a clay poultice to the back of neck about ½" thick and 3" by 6" in size. This will reduce headaches. Apply a clay poultice to your liver area about ½" thick and 10" in diameter. This is to aid in liver detox and rejuvenation.

Evening – Drink 6-8 ounces liquid Calcium Bentonite Clay. Do a full body Calcium Bentonite Clay wrap. Leave on for 45-60 minutes. Shower off.

Days 3-7

Morning – Drink 3 ounces Calcium Bentonite Clay liquid. Apply a clay poultice to the liver area. Take a clay bath.

Evening – Drink 3 ounces Calcium Bentonite Clay liquid. Take a clay bath.

Days 8-21

Morning – Drink 1 ounce liquid Calcium Bentonite Clay. Apply a clay poultice to the liver area. Take a clay bath.

Evening – Drink 1 ounce liquid Calcium Bentonite Clay.

ALLERGIES – HAY FEVER

Allergies and hay fever are caused by the release of histamines. The liver becomes plugged up with toxins and fatty tissue and therefore cannot produce the necessary antihistamines to neutralize the allergic reactions. The first thing to do is clean and rebuild the liver. Once that is done, the allergies and hay fever may disappear.

The good news about clay is that not only will it help stimulate the eliminatory channels, but also it can effectively treat allergies and hay fever. Adsorption is a relatively quick process – almost instantaneous in certain cases. The adsorptive surfaces of the clay prevent the allergic reaction by quickly neutralizing allergens before these foreign invaders can attach themselves to the blood cells. In addition, any histamines produced by the allergens that have "gotten away" can also be quickly adsorbed. Water-soluble allergens are bound up by the clay because of its intense hydrophilic (water-loving) nature.

Some people, after taking the clay, notice an immediate improvement in their conditions. Sometimes the allergies and hay fever disappear altogether. Others see no sudden improvement and must keep taking the clay quite a while before they obtain visible results. The reaction, of course, depends on the state of the liver and the condition of the immune system. A healthier liver will bounce back more quickly than one that is sick.

Allergy treatment with Calcium Bentonite Clay is as follows: (May be seasonal or ongoing)

Days 1-7

Morning – Drink 3 ounces liquid Calcium Bentonite Clay. Take a hot clay bath for 20 minutes. Apply a clay poultice to the liver area, approximately ½" thick and 10" in diameter.

Afternoon – Drink 3 ounces liquid Calcium Bentonite Clay.

Evening – Drink 3 ounces liquid Calcium Bentonite Clay. Apply a clay poultice to the liver area.

Days 8-21

Morning – Drink 1 ounce liquid Calcium Bentonite Clay. Take a 20-minute clay bath.

Afternoon – Drink 1 ounce liquid Calcium Bentonite Clay.

Evening – Drink 1 ounce liquid Calcium Bentonite Clay.

Days 21 + (Maintenance)

Drink 1-2 ounces liquid Calcium Bentonite Clay daily. Take 2-3 clay baths per week.

ALKALOSIS – see pH Balance

ANEMIA

Calcium Bentonite Clay is frequently used to stop anemia indirectly by increasing your red blood cell count. Clay's relationship to your liver and its ability to cleanse the liver is the action that causes it to produce more red blood cells. Anthropologists in various cultures around the world have observed the practice of using Calcium Bentonite Clay to cleanse and heal the liver, and in turn stop the anemia.

The following treatment is recommended for anemia:

When blood count is below normal:

Morning – Drink 3 ounces Calcium Bentonite Clay liquid. Apply a clay poultice over your liver area. Make the poultice approximately ½" thick and 10" in diameter. Leave on for about 30 minutes.

Evening – Drink 3 ounces Calcium Bentonite Clay liquid.

When blood count is normal but you have a history of anemia, continue the below regimen for 60 days.

Morning – Drink 2 ounces Calcium Bentonite Clay liquid.

Evening – Drink 2 ounces Calcium Bentonite Clay liquid.

ANOREXIA

Anorexia is a condition wherein you starve your body of food and, in turn, its necessary nutrients and vitamins. It is caused by an emotional disturbance which creates physical symptoms replicating starvation. While psychological counseling lies at the core of correcting the behaviors associated with this emotional disease, Calcium Bentonite Clay greatly aids the body in its recovery and restoration process. For an anorexic that is working to cure their disease, we recommend the following clay regimen in addition to food intake and psychological counseling:

Days 1-14

Morning – Drink 6 ounces liquid Calcium Bentonite Clay. Take a hot clay bath for 20 minutes.

Afternoon – Drink 6 ounces liquid Calcium Bentonite Clay.

Evening – Drink 6 ounces liquid Calcium Bentonite Clay.

Days 15-45 (until regular food intake is established)

Same as days 1-14, reducing liquid Calcium Bentonite Clay intake to 4 ounces on each occasion.

Days 45 + (Until optimal weight is reached)

Same as days 1-14, reducing liquid Calcium Bentonite Clay intake to 2 ounces on each occasion.

ARTHRITIS

Most arthritic conditions are due to an accumulation of waste matter, toxic by-product, that has settled in specific areas of the body such as the hands, knees, lower back, etc. Sometimes uric acid is the culprit and will attack the cartilage of the joints, the tendons, the ligaments, or other tissues, causing them to swell due to inflammation and toxic fluid buildup.

The clay's action is indirect in that it acts as an analgesic to reduce pain, an absorber of excess fluid buildup and a cleanser of toxicity. In turn the symptoms of arthritis disappear. Calcium Bentonite Clay will relieve the pain, reduce swelling and stiffness, and increase joint motion and range.

Try the following uses of clay to treat arthritis:

During presence of arthritic conditions:

Morning – Drink 2 ounces of liquid Calcium Bentonite Clay. Take a 20-minute hot clay bath. Pack the affected area thickly with hydrated Calcium Bentonite Clay and wrap loosely with a plastic wrap. Leave on for 1 hour.

Afternoon – Drink 2 ounces of liquid Calcium Bentonite Clay.

Evening – Drink 2 ounces of liquid Calcium Bentonite Clay. Put a thin film of hydrated Calcium Bentonite Clay on the affected areas. Leave on for a minimum of one hour. May be left on overnight.

Maintenance – No arthritic conditions present

Daily – Drink 1 ounce of liquid Calcium Bentonite Clay.

2-3 Times Weekly – Put a thin film of hydrated Calcium Bentonite Clay on the affected areas. Leave on for a minimum of one hour. May be left on overnight.

AUTISM

A leading national Calcium Bentonite Clay company has been working with two Autism clinics in the United States for the past 18 months. Through the use of Calcium Bentonite Clay baths, Autistic symptoms among children being treated through these clinics has dropped substantially.

It is believed that some of the varied contributory factors to autism range from aberrant brain wave transmission through the cerebral cortex, to food and environmental allergens, to metal toxicity. Each of these vastly different contributors, in fact all known variable factors contributing to autism, have one common denominator – a positive charged ionic base...and that is why clay is so very effective with autism.

Dr. Miriam Jang has seen many of her Autistic kids improving so much on the clay and she goes as far as saying that the clay works even better than the TD DMPS in chelation. "So far, I have put a huge number of patients on these clay baths and the levels of the heavy metals: mercury, lead, arsenic, aluminum and cadmium have come down dramatically. I follow the progress with 6 hour DMSA challenge urine test from Doctor's Data. One particular patient had very high levels of mercury and levels of lead that were off the charts. In 3 months of twice weekly clay baths, the lead came down dramatically and the mercury disappeared. The muscle weakness associated with high lead levels improved dramatically. Interestingly enough, another 5 months of these clay baths showed even lower levels of lead but the mercury re-appeared. This supports the theory that mercury is sequestered in different areas of our body and it takes time to get it all out."

According to Dr. Miriam Jang, the advantages of clay baths over TD DMPS and oral DMSA are:

a) "Almost zero side effects except drying of the skin which can be alleviated by a good moisturizer. You see, even though the TD DMPS is applied over the skin instead of ingested orally, there is still absorption of sulfur, which feeds the yeast and bad bacteria in the gut so that you can still have bad behaviors from the TD DMPS. I have quite a few patients that need to go on anti-fungals because of the TD DMPS. By the way, if your child is on TD DMPS and is irritable or hyper, please try adding lipoceutical glutathione. This has helped quite a few kids."

b) "No stress on the liver: clay baths do not elevate the liver enzymes, one less thing to worry about!"

c) "Cost: these clay baths are much less expensive compared to $150-$160 a bottle for TD DMPS or $95-$100 a bottle for DMSA."

d) "Ease of administration: It is dissolving a cup of powder clay in the bath and soaking for 15-30 minutes, twice a week. Most of our sweet Autistic kids love the bath anyway, so it really is not a bad way to get rid of metals."

e) "Faster results: I have been monitoring the levels of metals using all 3 methods and the clay baths are much faster in the removal of metals."

f) "Covers a wider spectrum of metals: For instance, DMSA and TD DMPS do not remove aluminum or nickel well. In addition, clay baths are good for environmental toxins so that we can start de-toxifying some of the chemicals that accumulate in our kids. I advocate the whole family doing these baths since we all have some accumulation."

The below treatment regimen is the one recommended by a leading Autism clinic.

Morning – Drink 2-3 ounces liquid Calcium Bentonite Clay.

Evening – Drink 2-3 ounces liquid Calcium Bentonite Clay.

3 Times Weekly – Take a clay bath in hot water for 20 minutes.

After 3 weeks reduce liquid to 1 ounce in morning and evening.

BAD BREATH

Clay has often been referred to as an internal mouthwash. That's because taking the clay daily will help to relieve the digestive tract, supporting elimination and binding the poisons that may be the cause of the unpleasant smell. This collection of poisons is likely the root of bad breath. Therefore, the channels of elimination must be activated. Once they are clean, there will be no bad odor to escape through the mouth.

For bad breath, brush your teeth and tongue with hydrated Calcium Bentonite Clay twice daily. Drink 2 ounces of liquid Calcium Bentonite Clay twice daily.

BEE STINGS – see Insect Stings

BIRTHMARK – see Lipofuscin Abnormalities

BLACKHEADS – see Acne

BLISTERS

All raised, fluid filled blisters are treated in exactly the same fashion. It matters not whether the blister was raised due to a burn, from breaking in a new shoe, or from too much gardening with no gloves. A blister, is a blister, is a blister. The treatment goal is threefold - First, to remove the pain, second, to remove the fluid without breaking the blister and third to leave no scar. All these are easily accomplished with use of Calcium Bentonite Clay.

The application is simple. Apply a thick gob of hydrated Calcium Bentonite Clay to the blister and surrounding 2" of skin. Cover that with plastic wrap. Leave it on until it begins to dry out, then wash off the old clay and reapply in the same fashion.

Pain should subside almost immediately. All of the fluid should be gone in 12-24 hours. And the healing process should be completed in 24-48 hours with no skin breakage or additional recovery time. At night, simply cover the affected area with clay and plastic, then pull on a piece of clothing such as a sock (if blister is on your foot) or a glove (glister on hand), etc., and go to sleep. Clean and redress in the morning.

BOILS

These badly infected pores are the result of an acne type of clogged pore becoming infected and not draining on its own. These large, postulates are oftentimes very painful and long lasting. Calcium Bentonite Clay is quite effective in healing boils. Often, if the boil has not yet come to a head, the clay will stop the degradation in its tracks and heal the developing boil in 1-2 days. If the boil has come to a head and may even have opened releasing pus and fluid, the healing process is quickened with use of Calcium Bentonite Clay. Try the following regime.

Days 1-2:

Morning – Drink 3 ounces of liquid Calcium Bentonite Clay. Prepare a poultice about ¼" thick and 4" in diameter to apply to the affected area.

Apply for 30-45 minutes.

Afternoon – Repeat morning process.

Evening – Repeat morning process.

Days 3-4 (or until boil is completely healed)

Same as days 1-2 treatment but reducing liquid Calcium Bentonite Clay drink to 1 ounce, three times a day.

BREAST HEALTH – see Cancer and Pregnancy

BROKEN BONES

Calcium Bentonite Clay speeds the healing time of broken bones to half of the normal course of events. In addition to the direct benefit of the Calcium mineral in the clay, it also reduces swelling, acts as a pain reducer and brings circulation to the affected area.

Recommendation for broken bones is internal and topical.

Days 1-7

Morning – Drink 2 ounces Calcium Bentonite Clay liquid. If possible, cut a hole in the cast and lay a cloth with clay on it in the hold. Another option is to make warm clay poultice packs in large 1-gallon ziplock bags. Lay these on the outside of the cast for 30-45 minutes.

Afternoon – Drink 2 ounces Calcium Bentonite Clay liquid.

Evening – Repeat morning process.

Days 8 – until cast removed or bone healed

Same as days 1-7 except reduce liquid Calcium Bentonite Clay from 2 ounces to 1 ounce, three times a day.

Apply a thin coating of hydrated clay topically after the cast is removed to assist with rebuilding tissue and strengthening the bones.

BROWN RECLUSE SPIDER BITE – see Spider Bites 43

BRUISES

Calcium Bentonite Clay is effective on any size bruise on any part of your body. Living Clay reduces the pain, removes the old fluid from the bruised area and restores new healthy circulation to the area.

Days 1-2

Morning – Drink 2 ounces Calcium Bentonite Clay liquid. For small bruises, apply a thin coat of hydrated clay to the area. Allow to dry then wash off. For larger bruises, apply a poultice, about ¼" thick and a little larger in diameter than the bruise. Leave on for 45-60 minutes.

Afternoon – Repeat morning treatment.

Evening – Drink 2 ounces Calcium Bentonite Clay liquid. Apply a thin coat of hydrated Calcium Bentonite Clay and leave on overnight.

Days 3-5 (until bruise is gone)

Repeat protocol from days 1-2, and reduce liquid Calcium Bentonite Clay to 1 ounce, three times a day.

BUNIONS – see Corns

BURNS

Burns coated with clay heal better, more rapidly and leave less scarring than other methods, especially if the clay is applied immediately.

Apply cold clay, in thick poultices, to the entire burn area. Reapply wet poultices until tenderness is gone.

Clay reduces all risks of infection and absorbs all the impurities and foreign bodies apt to be found in the burn. It also eliminates the destroyed cells, enabling cellular rebuilding.

Throughout the burn healing process drink one ounce of Calcium Bentonite Clay liquid, 3 times daily.

Renew the poultice application day and night, changing them every hour, until the appearance of new tissue occurs. Then reduce the frequency of application, but not to less than 3 or 4 poultices a day, and leave the poultices in place for two hours each, until the tissues are virtually rebuilt.

If the burns are on the feet or hands, dip them directly into a container of hydrated clay paste. It is necessary to remain immersed for an hour so that no trace of the burn will remain on completion of this mud bath. For extended area burns, it is advisable to coat the whole body with clay. Do not forget all other measures for maintaining a general healthy state.

CALLUSES AND CRACKED HEELS

The important thing for calluses, as well as dry cracked heels, is to re-moisturize, soften, and bring new circulation to the affected area. Both are treated with liquid Calcium Bentonite Clay and topical applications of hydrated Calcium Bentonite Clay.

Drink 1 ounce of liquid Calcium Bentonite Clay 3 times daily for treatment of any type of callus.

For small or localized calluses, cover the area with a thick application of hydrated Calcium Bentonite Clay, cover with plastic and leave on for 1 hour. Repeat this process 3 times daily until healed.

For cracked and possibly bleeding heels: In the morning, apply a relatively thick coating of hydrated Calcium Bentonite Clay. Cover with a large piece of plastic wrap such as Glad Press n' Seal. Then pull a sock over the wrap and wear for 2-3 hours. Repeat the process in the evening and leave on overnight for quicker results.

An ideal method is to soak the foot in a warm clay bath by diluting 1-2 cups of hydrated clay with one cup of warm water. Soak the foot for 30 minutes to an hour. Repeat daily. Corns and calluses tend to peel off. This hard to treat problem is often solved in as little as 3-4 days.

CANCER

"You've got cancer…" That's the most dreaded diagnosis in our world today. It's the way out of this lifetime we fear most.

The word "malignant" is an English word, not Latin as is the case with many disease names, and when translated it means "rapidly reproducing, positive ionic charged cells, which we as doctors haven't yet figured out how to contain, and they scare us to death, literally."

Fortunately, for all of us, Calcium Bentonite Clay, which is a strongly negative charged ionic molecule, is blind and has no fears. It's been running down dark alleys chasing positive charged ions for centuries, rounding them up and "saving" bodies from their ravages. It's all in a day's work for Calcium Bentonite Clay. In many cases Calcium Bentonite Clay has also helped in discarding dead cells from the body following chemo and radiation treatments. The problem lies in difficult to reach regions of the body. Ideally, daily ingestion of Calcium Bentonite Clay is a great preventative measure for cancers, as acidic environments are breeding grounds for the rapid reproduction of cancer cells. Calcium Bentonite Clay's high pH helps brings the body into balance and reduces acidic conditions. In some cases, Living Clay can assist the body in restoring health by eliminating highly toxic conditions.

And before we go any further, here's a word from our friends at the FDA: "As with all major, life threatening ailments, we encourage you to consult with your doctor before altering any treatment program you are now on. Your condition may be so advanced, your body so ill, that you may do further harm by altering your current treatment. No statement we make, or information we offer, should be construed as a claim for a cure, treatment or prevention of any disease." Thank you for listening...

All forms of cancer should be attacked in the same fashion - aggressively. Whether it be a blood borne type such as leukemia, a lymph glad or tumorous carcinogen such as breast cancer, an organ specific cancer such as prostate cancer, or something as "simple" as a small nodule of skin cancer – a full frontal attack is warranted. Cancers are the craftiest of all cells, having the ability to multiply a thousand fold in minutes as well as to mutate into various other forms of its ilk.

Shown below is the broadest of outlines as to how to deal with various cancers. You might consider consulting with or visiting one of the several treatment centers across the United States using Calcium Bentonite Clay to remove cancerous cells. These are excellent medical facilities and have such things as Calcium Bentonite Clay immersion pits available for ease of treatment. They are also familiar with traditional modalities of treatment and can best assist you in making decisions regarding your health.

Use of liquid Calcium Bentonite Clay – When attacking cancer cells, drink 6-8 ounces of liquid Calcium Bentonite Clay three times daily. Continue this practice until in complete remission. Then maintain a regimen of 1 ounce twice daily as a lifetime practice. I have heard from people who drink as much as a quart of liquid Calcium Bentonite Clay per day. Remember, Calcium Bentonite Clay can do no harm. Learn to listen to your body. It will instruct you on proper dosage and how much it requires.

Clay Baths – We recommend a minimum of one clay bath per day until in remission. Use double the normal amount of clay. Use one half-gallon liquid Calcium Bentonite Clay or 16 ounces of dry powder in every bath. Upon remission continue to treat yourself to one Calcium Bentonite Clay bath per week for general health purposes.

Clay Poultices – If you have a localized tumor, cancerous lumps or mass, or localized skin cancer, use poultices on a regular basis. A poultice can be anywhere from ¼" to 1" thick and from 2" to 12" in diameter. It could be referred to as a "clay patty," similar to those "mud patties" you played with as a child. (You didn't know it then, but you were in training...) Place the clay patty on a large piece of cloth/gauze/plastic and apply over the mass. Leave on for 30-60 minutes. Repeat this process several times a day, using a new batch of clay for each poultice.

47

Clay Suppositories – Mix some thick clay paste and form into suppository shaped "bullets." We're goin' cancer hunting! Allow to dry in open air until very firm or actually dry. Then simply rewet the surface for easy insertion. For prostate cancer, uterine cancer, any cancer, which is directly accessible through one of our "dark alleys" referred to earlier, use suppositories to get up close and personal for best effectiveness. If used vaginally, douche to remove residue.

Hydrated Clay Wraps – One of the most effective uses of Calcium Bentonite Clay is the clay immersion pit. If one is not available to you, the next best thing is a full body clay wrap – from head to toe – everything but the whites of your eyes and ear canals.

After applying the clay either stand in open air until it dries then shower off, or wrap yourself gently in plastic wrap or towels to slow the drying process and extend the treatment to an hour or more. Then shower off and towel dry.

One other factor to be aware of regarding cancers – all cancers – cancers <u>require</u> an acidic environment to multiply and flourish. Calcium Bentonite Clays have a pH as high as 9.7 – extremely alkaline. Calcium Bentonite Clay raises your body's pH, removes positive charged ions, cleanses and detoxes as it does its work. Calcium Bentonite Clay is cancer's worst natural nightmare…

CANDIDA

Treat as follows:

Morning – Drink 3 ounces liquid Calcium Bentonite Clay. For females, insert vaginally one Calcium Bentonite Clay suppository. Leave in 2 hours then douche to remove residue. Take a clay bath for 20 minutes.

Afternoon – Drink 3 ounces liquid Calcium Bentonite Clay.

Evening – Drink 3 ounces liquid Calcium Bentonite Clay.

If you have a lifetime history of Candida reoccurrences, maintain a regimen as follows:

Morning – Drink 2 ounces liquid Calcium Bentonite Clay.

Twice a Week – Take a clay bath.

CARPEL TUNNEL SYNDROME

Clay for Carpel Tunnel syndrome is a simple process and relief occurs in as little as 1 day. Use as follows:

Drink 1 ounce liquid Calcium Bentonite Clay twice daily.

Prepare hydrated Calcium Bentonite Clay warmed wraps and wrap completely around the wrists. Make the wraps about ¼" – ½" thick. Cover with plastic wrap and leave on overnight. This will have a tremendous effect on Carpel Tunnel Syndrome, usually within 48 hours.

Some people have reported increased localized pain and stiffness after their first night's application. However, these same people then have reported a lessening of pain after 48 hours, and complete relief after 72 hours. Full motor control, in the most severe cases I've seen, is usually regained within three weeks of continued treatment. In two people that I've seen, the pain began to return two months later; one treatment of clay relieved all newly occurring pain.

How can clay possibly accomplish this? The answer is as simple as it is mysterious. In his article "True Carpal Tunnel Syndrome" (Paul R. Martin, McHenry NeuroDiagnonstics, McHenry, Illinois, Copyright 1996) Paul writes, "Anything which will promote circulation, help to relieve inflammation, aid in removal of local toxins, and soothe irritated muscles and tendons will help Carpal Tunnel Syndrome."

Healing clay packs work energetically with the human system. By actually pulling contaminants through the skin (due to its electromagnet properties), the clay reduces swelling and inflammation and STIMULATES the immune system. The energy exchange that occurs in a Calcium Bentonite Clay action is so evident that it can be visually measured, oftentimes in only days.

CATARACTS

Cataracts are the result of localized buildups of positive charged ions, which occur in and on the eye itself. Successful removal and return of 20/20 sight has been reported using Calcium Bentonite Clay in the following fashion:

Morning – Drink 2 ounces liquid Calcium Bentonite Clay. Apply a packed telfa pad over a closed eyelid (as you would a slice of cucumber) and leave on for 1 hour. Do not put Calcium Bentonite Clay directly on the exposed eyeball as it has a drying effect, which is not good for the moisture needed for your eyes. You may also apply hydrated Calcium Bentonite

Clay in a thin film on your eyelid and surrounding area as would be done in a facial. Allow it to dry, then wash off.

Afternoon – repeat morning process.

Evening – repeat morning process.

CELLULOSE – see Weight Loss

CHEMOTHERAPY DETOXIFICATION
Post-Chemotherapy Care, Treatment & Detox

Clay Therapy, both internal and external, during the crucial rest time between chemotherapy treatments is important. This detox strategy will assist the patient to recover and stabilize in time for the next treatment. After the chemotherapy treatments are finished the critical convalescing period begins.

It should be noted that Calcium Bentonite Clay might allow some patients to complete the series of chemotherapy treatment that would otherwise withdraw before completion. This is where Calcium Bentonite Clay goes head-on against the dangerous accumulation of toxic waste and all the debilitating attending side effects.

Examples of this detox/healing process will start with topical oral hygiene: gums, mouth sores, tongue, lips, throat, etc. External will be the obvious skin problems: infection, fungus, yeast infection, etc.

Full Body Wraps – Daily with slightly warmed clay. Put some clay in a zip lock bag and put the bag in a sink of warm water for a few minutes. Apply to full body, head to toe, and allow to dry in a warm room. Even a partial treatment, such as face or neck, upper or lower body, or only legs and feet would be of value to the stressed patient. But a "full-body" treatment will be an exceptional and favored tactic to dramatically reduce the incapacitating flood of toxic poisoning that is overwhelming and literally choking the patient's system. Wrap in a sheet if necessary while drying.

Detox Clay Bath – Pour two cups of liquid clay in hot bath water. After a full body wrap soak in a clay bath or just as a bath soak. Or you can sprinkle in one to two cups of powdered clay and swish around as the bath water is filling. Soak for no more than 20 minutes.

Clay Drink – Drink Liquid Clay, 4 ounces, three times a day. Mix the liquid Calcium Bentonite Clay with juice or in a glass of water. Drink water during the day as well. Drinking Calcium Bentonite Clay is also good for settling and balancing a toxic, nauseous stomach, acid reflux, and stopping diarrhea.

Calcium Bentonite Clay suppositories for detox and healing research will include hemorrhoid, vaginal and anal fistula treatments, along with feminine hygiene needs. Take some hydrated clay and mix a little powder with it to firm it into a workable consistency. Form into bullet shaped suppositories and allow to dry slightly until firm enough to insert as a suppository. Rewet to lubricate for insertion.

The cancer chemotherapy patient is in dire need of the detoxification and wound healing, soothing properties of Calcium Bentonite Clay. Their whole system has been in a physical, emotional, chemical wreck, is totally exhausted, and full of poison.

Antibiotics are of little or no value. Their immune system is desperately depressed and in overload. It just can't deal with the bacterial and toxic assault.

The body needs help to absorb and adsorb the mass of toxins and poisonous waste that one's system wasn't designed to handle. The ailing body needs assistance in searching out, capturing, and removing the destructive bacteria, which are growing by a billion or so every hour.

It seems that clay has, among other properties, the ability to stimulate a deficiency or absorb an excess of the radioactivity in the body. On an organism that has suffered and still retains the radiations of radium (or any other intensive radioactive source), the radioactivity is first enhanced and then absorbed. Clay could, in this way, ensure the protection of organisms over-exposed to atomic radiations. This radioactive effect has been researched: today, when everyone is forcibly submitted to many artificially provoked radioactive aggressions, such as dust in the atmosphere from bomb testing, everything increasing this danger should be avoided. Experiments made with the Geiger encounter have demonstrated that dry Calcium Bentonite Clay absorbs a very important part of this surrounding radioactivity.

Clay can absorb/adsorb infection in tissue/blood, and acts as nature's referee so your body can heal itself.

Remember, Calcium Bentonite Clay can't be used wrong. Drink it, put it on your body, and bathe in it.

CHEMICAL BURNS – see Burns

CHRONIC FATIGUE SYNDROME (CFS)

Recent research from Temple University suggests that a blood marker from chronic fatigue syndrome (CFS) may soon be available. Researchers have isolated a specific antiviral pathway that consistently demonstrates disruption in immune function.

A low-density enzyme unique to people with CFS is the suspected culprit. With chronic fatigue syndrome, RNA (ribonucleic acid) function in the body becomes disrupted, inhibiting protein synthesis. This causes various symptoms, such as tiredness, aches and pains, delayed muscle recovery, and mood swings. CFS is referred to as a complex illness, because of the many symptoms it produces.

Proper rest is essential to the successful treatment of CFS, but the right balance of activity is also crucial. Absolute inactivity can result in a deconditioned state. On the other hand, becoming too active may overextend the muscles, thus delaying chances for recovery. Therefore, people with this condition must avoid strenuous activity and must treat the sleep disorder, so common in this condition that may further aggravate the muscle pain.

People with this disorder must take a host-centered approach to the illness: stimulating the bodies own forces of healing though lifestyle changes to bring about recovery. Detoxification is obviously needed. Since immune function is governed by the Kupffer cells of the liver, which in turn respond to the chemical balance of the colon, rebalancing the chemical state of the colon is necessary. In other words, keeping the gut clear will assist in combating the degenerative effects of the disease. Calcium Bentonite Clay should be taken daily to adsorb bodily toxins and ensure intestinal health.

Often several viruses and fungi are activated in cases of CFS. For instance, many people who come down with the illness are diagnosed with Candida in the gut. According to an article in the *Canadian Journal of Microbiology*, clay has the capacity to adsorb and eliminate viruses (Lipson an Stolzky 1985).

Taking Calcium Bentonite Clay internally has many advantages, one being its ability to act as a pattern and catalyst for the formation of long peptide chains. The ability to form peptide chains is one of the keys to increasing immuno ability, which lies at the crux of the cause of CFS.

Drink liquid Calcium Bentonite Clay in the amount of 3 ounces, three times per day, and taking 3-4 clay baths per week. In addition, 2 full body wraps per week will quicken the healing process.

Ridding your body of CFS can be an extended process. Symptomatic relief can be experienced in as little as 3-5 days, but complete remission of the ailment may take 2-3 months.

COLD SORES – see Herpes Virus

COLON CLEANSE

When discussing a colon cleanse, I think we should broaden our view to the aspect of an Internal Cleanse of the entire digestive tract. While it is true that a colon cleanse may be accomplished with clay colonics and drinking liquid Calcium Bentonite Clay, we will cover every aspect of an internal cleanse from the mouth, south. In this day and age, we ALL need to cleanse!

"In a world where dietary choices are poor, environmental pollution is heavy, stress levels are high, and exercise is often a last priority, **internal cleansing is more important than ever** for optimum health." ~ Dr. Bernard Jensen

Understanding the basics of how our digestive system works is vital to understanding personal health. Before we can fully grasp the extreme importance of internal cleansing, we must first know what's going on in there. So, let's start with a quick primer on the digestive system.

54   Dr. Lindsey Duncan, CN, ND, provides the following succinct tutorial:

> We live and die by what foods we put in our mouth and how our bodies assimilate these foods. Digestion starts in our mouths, when we bite into our food and begin chewing it and mixing it with saliva, a powerful digestive enzyme. As our food travels down to the stomach, it mixes with hydrochloric acid, a powerful digestive acid that liquefies the food and prepares it for further digestion in the small intestines with help from the pancreas and liver.
>
> Our intestinal systems are connected to a network of blood vessels and veins, which wrap around the stomach, small intestine, and bowel. Our blood receives nutrients from our digested food through this network of blood vessels, which look and function much like the roots of a tree, drawing dissolved nutrients out of the intestines and transporting them to the liver, where they undergo further breakdown, recombination, and storage. Later, the heart pumps

these nutrients, stored in the liver, to nourish the various living cells that make up the tissues of the human body. By-products of the digestive process are passed into the bowel, where they solidify, and "in a perfect world," are completely excreted from the body.

This is basically how our body gets nourishment and energy. After it delivers nutrients throughout the body, the blood also collects cellular waste materials (by-products of metabolism) and "drops them off" at appropriate eliminative stations (lung, kidneys, skin, lymphatic system, colon) where, also, "in a perfect world" they are quickly excreted from the body.

Unfortunately, our "modern day society" is NOT a perfect world. Pollutants, toxins, chemicals, fertilizers, growth hormones, pesticides and other hazards to our health bombard and infiltrate our air, water and food on a daily basis. Our diets, no longer wholesome and fresh, consist of fast foods, junk foods, pre-prepared foods, fatty foods, and devitalized foods. There is no way our digestive systems can function optimally with the heavy burdens placed on them on a day-to-day basis. Digestion becomes sluggish, assimilation becomes inefficient, mal-absorption of nutrients begins, the metabolism slows down (weight gain!) and elimination becomes poor.

A clean, properly functioning bowel is paramount to our well being. Dr. Bernard Jensen, nutritionist, lecturer and author of over 30 books on natural health care, states this best:

"Every cell and tissue in the body is fed by the bloodstream, which is supplied by the bowel. When the bowel is dirty, the blood is dirty and so are the organs and tissues. It is the bowel that must be cared for first before any effective healing can take place."

So, how do you know the state of your bowels? How do you know if you need to do an internal cleanse? Dr. Duncan writes:

"Many of my seminar topics focus on internal cleansing and bowel management. Repeatedly, I am asked the same question by seminar attendees: "How do I know if I need to cleanse?" My answer is quite simple... After consulting with over 20,000 patients, I can honestly state that I have never worked with an individual that did not directly benefit from detoxifying his or her body. **In this day and age, we ALL need to cleanse!** In a world where dietary choices are poor, environmental pollution is heavy, stress levels are high, and exercise is often a last priority, **internal cleansing is more important than ever** for optimum health."

Okay, I get it. I need to cleanse, you need to cleanse, EVERYBODY needs to cleanse! How is it done, and what should be used? According to Ran Knishinsky, author of The Clay Cure, *the best, most natural way to internally cleanse is with Calcium Bentonite Clay. The following is an excerpt from his book:*

If the system fails to get rid of poisons through the bowels, a constipated condition arises in which the toxins never leave the body. They sit inside and putrefy. What's worse, the body doesn't know the difference between live food and dead food in the colon. It will still try to get nourishment out of waste you would never want to set your eyes upon. Naturally, this puts a strain on every functioning cell in the body.

Calcium Bentonite Clay's immediate action upon the body is directly on the digestive channel. This involves the clay actually binding with the toxic substances and removing them from the body with the stool. It performs this job with every kind of toxin, including those from the environment, such as heavy metals, and those that occur naturally as by-products of the body's own health processes, such as metabolic toxins. It's hard to believe that the body produces its own toxins, but that may happen as a result of stress, inefficient metabolism, or the proliferation of free radicals.

The body has no problem ridding itself of the clay. Don't worry about a tiny brick house being built in the middle of your colon. The clay assists the body's eliminatory process by acting as a bulking agent, similar to psyllium fiber, sweeping out the old matter that doesn't need to be there. It is not digested in the same manner as food as it passes through the alimentary canal. Instead, it stimulates intestinal peristalsis, the muscular contractions that move food and stool through the bowels. The clay and the adsorbed toxins are both eliminated together; this keeps the toxins from being reabsorbed into the bloodstream.

Clay works on the entire organism. No one part of the body is left untouched by its healing energies. I don't know of another supplement that is quite as capable as clay of producing such a wide range of positive reactions."

Our Recommendations for Internal Cleansing

Ran Knishinsky recommends ingesting clay on a daily basis to maintain optimal health. I agree, and offer several ways you can do this.

For internal cleansing, you must ingest clay. You have several options for doing so: you can eat hydrated clay, drink liquefied clay or stir powder clay into a glass of water and drink. If you choose to eat clay, hydrated clay has a thick, smooth consistency. Generally, it is suggested that one to two tablespoons of hydrated clay daily is the proper amount for an adult. For those who prefer to take their clay in liquid form, start with one to two ounces of Calcium Bentonite Clay Liquid daily. If you've never tasted Calcium Bentonite Clay Liquid, you should know that it has a very creamy smooth consistency, and is virtually tasteless. It is recommended to take the clay on an empty stomach for best results. And if you're taking any medication, it is recommended to wait 1-4 hours before ingesting clay, but please check with your physician, as medications vary in time release and content.

People who have made this a part of their daily routine have been astounded with the outcome. According to Knishinsky, benefits reported by people using liquid clay for a period of two to four weeks include: improved intestinal regularity; relief from chronic constipation, diarrhea, indigestion, and ulcers; a surge in physical energy; clearer complexion; brighter, whiter eyes; enhanced alertness; emotional uplift; improved tissue and gum repair; and increased resistance to infections. Clay works on the entire organism. No part of the body is left untouched by its healing energies.

So, begin your internal cleansing program today. Ingesting Calcium Bentonite Clay on a daily basis will get your intestines clean, and keep them that way! Make Calcium Bentonite Clay a part of your daily routine, and experience all the life-enhancing benefits that Calcium Bentonite Clay has to give!

COLON POLYPS - see Colon Cleanse

CONSTIPATION

When the bowels do not move properly, the reasons are usually improper diet, lack of fiber, lack of water, and faulty digestion. The first thing to do is drink lots of water – no other liquids, just water. That will help the Calcium Bentonite Clay to work and get the system normalized.

Clay produces desirable bulk in the intestinal tract, which in turn stimulates normal intestinal motions and contractions that move food substances in the intestine. Therefore, it can help protect against chronic constipation. Clay is not a laxative, however. Laxatives work by irritating the mucous membranes, causing the colon to contract.

Begin taking the clay once a day on an empty stomach before retiring to bed. Allow the clay at least one to seven days to regulate the system; thereafter, eat it on a maintenance dose.

A word to the wise: If you drink an adequate amount of water when taking the clay, the constipation will likely be eased in 2 days. We suggest 2-3 ounces of the liquid clay, three times per day until regular. Follow that with daily maintenance doses of 1-2 ounces as a lifetime practice.

CORNS AND BUNIONS

Corns and bunions are treated in the same fashion as calluses and cracked heels. Some can be healed in as little as 3-4 days and in most all cases, no more than 2-3 weeks no matter how bad or how old the corn or bunion. Treat as follows:

First, remove the stimulus, which caused the problem in the first place, such as shoes that are too tight.

Secondly, drink 1 ounce liquid Calcium Bentonite Clay 3 times daily until the problem is completely gone.

Third, prepare a small poultice, or hydrated Calcium Bentonite Clay pad, to completely cover the corn/bunion and the surrounding area. Cover with plastic wrap. Change this poultice pad 3 to 4 times daily and leave one on at bedtime. Change the next morning.

After the corn/bunion is completely gone, maintain 1 ounce liquid Calcium Bentonite Clay daily as a lifetime practice.

CRACKED HEELS - see Calluses

CRAMPS – see Muscle Soreness/Cramps

CUTS

For treatment of an open, bleeding cut, pack clay powder directly into the wound to stop the bleeding. After bleeding has clotted or stopped, rinse the cut with cool water and repack with powder clay or apply a cool poultice. Cover the area to keep clean.

After this poultice, which should be kept in place for a maximum of 2 hours, wash the wound with water, and apply a compress of clayish water.

If the existence of foreign bodies in the wound is feared, continue the clay poultices until there is no more doubt. All the foreign substances will be adsorbed and pulled from the body by the clay. There have been many cases where foreign bodies that were difficult to extract surgically have been drawn out by the clay.

When the state of the wound allows it, expose it to the open air in order to hasten its healing. Sometimes it is necessary to apply a dry dressing in order to avoid friction or direct contact with the wound.

To avoid this, keep the wound lightly covered in hydrated clay. If ever a bandage sticks to a cut or wound, simply hold under running water until the bandage pulls itself away.

Cuts heal in half the normal time, using clay as the healing agent. Clay also greatly reduces the possibility of scarring after healing has occurred.

CYSTS – see Tumors

DANDRUFF
Dandruff is easily managed with daily use of Calcium Bentonite Clay. Use as follows:

Days 1-7

Morning – Drink 3 ounces of liquid Calcium Bentonite Clay. "Shampoo" hair with hydrated Calcium Bentonite Clay. Apply to all of head as you would a thick cream rinse. Leave on for 5-10 minutes. Rinse off thoroughly

Evening – Drink 3 ounces of liquid Calcium Bentonite Clay.

Days 8-21

Drink 1 ounce of liquid Calcium Bentonite Clay twice daily. "Shampoo" hair daily as described above.

After dandruff is gone and no traces remain, continue a daily lifetime practice of drinking one ounce of liquid Calcium Bentonite Clay and shampooing hair with hydrated Calcium Bentonite Clay as necessary. Follow with a cream rinse.

DEPRESSION – see Detoxification - Full Body (Shown Below)

Cleansing and detoxing your body as a first step can best help emotional disturbances.

DETOXIFICATION – FULL BODY

There is no single treatment of more value to the human body than a complete full body detoxification protocol using Calcium Bentonite Clay as the cleansing agent and carrier for toxin removal.

The great majority of articles on detox and colon cleansing should be classified as colon cleansers themselves, because they will most certainly scare the poo right out of you! They explain how substances that are toxic to our bodies come at us from all directions: the air we breathe, the food we eat, the water we drink, the cleaning products we use, and the metabolic waste produced inside us. Studies have discovered various chemicals from our foods and environment that indicate man contributes 700,000 tons of pollutants into the air every day, ranging from everyday household cleaners to cosmetics and hair sprays. That's just the air! Add in the pesticides and toxins that are found in our water. Don't forget the chemicals that are routinely fed to the animals we eat, and the sprayed, preserved, and genetically altered plants we consume. And that doesn't even factor in the heavy metal poisoning that's occurring at a truly alarming rate - from the lead in our paint to the mercury in the fish we eat and the fillings in our teeth, and everything in between. It's truly frightening. The reports are everywhere.

You can spend weeks reading article after article, complete with pictures that will keep you awake at night. We, however, want you to rest easy. We have chosen, therefore, to concentrate on **the benefits of detox - to emphasize the positive** instead of beating you over the head with the all too prevalent negative. Granted, what we've done to our bodies and our environment is truly frightening, and the state of our digestive systems - and consequently our health in general - is nightmarish because of it. Enough said. Now, here's the good stuff!

The Benefits of Detoxification

Science has shown that the effects of detoxification on our body's cells are nothing short of **miraculous**. The following is an excerpt from Natasha Lee's article "Could Detoxification be the Fountain of Youth?

"Dr. Alexis Carrel, of the Rockefeller Institute for Medical Research performed an amazing experiment in the early 1900's. He managed to sustain the life of cells from a chicken embryo by immersing it in a solution containing all the nutrients necessary for life and changing the solution daily. The cells took up nutrients from the nutrient-rich broth and excreted their wastes into the same solution. The only thing Dr. Carrel did each day was discard the old solution and replace it with fresh nutrient solution. The chicken cells lived for **29 years** until one night Dr. Carrel's assistant forgot to change the polluted solution! We do not know how much longer the cell's life could have been maintained.

Dr. Carrel concluded at the end of his experiment that **the cell is actually immortal. It is merely the fluid in which it floats which degenerates**. He is quoted saying, "The cell is immortal, renew this fluid at intervals, give the cell something on which to feed and, so far as we know, the pulsation of life may go on forever." The average chicken lives about 7 years. His detoxified, properly nourished chicken cell lived for 29 years.

It may be hard to believe that the body could live indefinitely, however, a similar level of vibrant health and life extension can be created in humans by following the obvious similar principal.

Every cell in our body excretes waste material, which becomes toxic, and poisonous to our bodies if we allow it to build up faster than we renew the fluid in which it floats. According to the above experiment, **this is the cause of aging and degeneration**. Factors such as "time" and ideas such as "that's just life" fade from the picture, with new data in view. The fact is, **every 7 years we have a completely new set of bones, teeth, skin and hair**. Logically, a person should be able to look and feel better than they did 7 years ago by changing and improving the way they take care of their own body as Dr. Carrel took care of his chicken cell.

Time alone is not a disease or poison, it is the toxins that accumulate with time that the body cannot withstand and so deteriorates from. In other words, time alone is not the cause of death. Poisons are the cause of death of life forms.

So, logically and from the above data **by detoxifying your cells a person can freshen up and grow healthier and younger than they once were** by practicing this principle. Periodically detoxifying the body, drinking lots of fresh water and staying smart on nutrition can appear to work miracles. Dr. Carrel however proved these amazing results are not miracles, just good science."

Kathryn Alexander, one of the leading experts in detoxification and dietary healing states it succinctly; "The legacy of 50 years exposure to persistent man-made chemicals combined with the denigration of the food chain has increased our susceptibility to chronic degenerative disease and cancer. Reversal can only come about by resolving these primary causes of disease. **By releasing the toxic burden of the body and restoring its nutritional status, we can change our internal environment and achieve good health.**"

The most common symptom of autointoxication (self-poisoning caused by endogenous microorganisms, metabolic wastes, or other toxins produced within the body) is mental dullness and fatigue. Other common symptoms are headache, constipation, diarrhea, colds, general aches and pains, particularly up and down the spine and especially in the low back, skin problems, common infections (due to lowered immunocompetence), morning sluggishness, gas, bad breath, foulsmelling stool, allergies, intolerance to fatty foods, premenstrual tension, breast soreness and tendency to repeated vaginal infections. The good news...Detoxification can relieve these symptoms!

Using Calcium Bentonite Clay to Detox

So, how do we go about this detox business? The answer is simple - **CLAY**! Not just any clay, but Calcium Bentonite Clay. A recognized detoxifying agent, it is in the Smectite group of clays. **Only those clays within the Smectite group have the ability to absorb as well as adsorb**. This means that as the clay passes through your body, it's negative ionic charge will draw to it anything with· a positive charge (bacteria, viruses, toxins, etc.) and will remove them from your body. The clay adsorbs (positively charged particles are drawn to, and stick to it's surface) and also absorbs these particles. The clay passes through your body, and the toxins are removed as waste.

Ran Knishinsky, author of *The Clay Cure*, is an advocate of eating or drinking clay daily. In his book, he states some of the benefits reported by people using liquid clay for a period of two to four weeks include: improved intestinal regularity; relief from chronic constipation, diarrhea, indigestion, and ulcers; a surge in physical energy; clearer complexion; brighter, whiter eyes; enhanced alertness; emotional uplift; improved tissue and gum repair; and increased resistance to infections. Calcium Bentonite Clay works on the entire organism. No part of the body is left untouched by its healing energies.

We recommend taking clay daily to maintain a good, clean digestive system. Normal amounts for adults to take are as follows: Liquid Clay - 1 to 6 ounces daily, Hydrated Clay - 1 to 2 Tablespoons daily. So, choose your method (liquid or hydrated) and stick with it! When taking clay internally, it is very important to keep the body hydrated by drinking 8 to 10 glasses of water daily. The water helps to soften and loosen impacted fecal material lining the walls of the small intestine and colon. This material is then absorbed by the clay and removed from the body through normal elimination.

To do a detox, however, higher doses are recommended. We suggest doubling the standard, maintenance doses listed above, by taking the clay in the morning, in the afternoon, and in the evening, preferably on an empty stomach. And if you're taking any medication, it is recommended to wait 1-3 hours before ingesting clay, but please check with your physician, as medications vary in time release and content. Also, Clay Baths are highly beneficial for detoxification, especially for cases of heavy metal poisoning. The directions for Clay Baths are listed below:

Clay Bath Directions for Detoxifying

Pour up to 2 cups of powdered clay in the bathtub and then run **very hot water** over the clay, as hot as it gets. Use a whisk or your hand to stir the clay around and to help it dissolve. When you've got about 3 inches of water in the tub and the clay is dissolved, start adding cooler water until the water reaches the desired temperature.

The bath should neither be too hot nor too cool, but should be nice and warm, as warm as is comfortable. Bathing time depends upon your condition, but can be anywhere from 15 to 20 minutes. **Please don't overdo it!** If you stay in too long there is a small possibility you could experience what is known as a cleansing reaction and feel fatigue, headaches, muscle soreness, etc. Be aware of your body's response to the first detox bath.

Another option is to take about 2 cups of extra thick liquid Calcium Bentonite Clay and put it into the bath water.

Others have used a full quart and more. It is highly effective in drawing out toxins. But too much, or too long exposure, may dry out the skin. If so, when necessary, follow the bath with a body lotion.

In *Energy to Heal*, by Wendell Hoffman, through his own research, Hoffman found that clean, natural Calcium Bentonite Clay used in a bath could actually **draw out toxic chemicals through the pores of the skin.** After many experiments, he concluded that optimum results are obtained by immersing oneself in a tub of very warm water mixed with a clean, natural Calcium Bentonite Clay for exactly 20 minutes! Not just any clay will do. It is crucial to use "clean clay."

Extreme amounts of clay used in a bath have been known to help the body detox from severe heavy metal poisoning. Usually 1 bath, 2-4 times in a week is sufficient to draw out the toxins.

Healing clays have been used for detoxification purposes for centuries and, due to several key factors, are irreplaceable as a part of a cleansing protocol.

"One of the most amazing effects of clay baths in particular is the ability of the clay to stimulate the lymphatic system. The more clay that is used in the therapy, the more powerful the response. I know of people who take clay baths in pits containing 1.5 tons of heated green Calcium Bentonite Clay." Jason Eaton, Eyton's Earth

Jason went on to say, "Fairly recently, I had the opportunity to meet with an individual who likely had one of the worst cases of environmental toxicity in the U.S. medical history. He eventually found treatment at the John Hopkins Center for Environmental Medicine, under the care of Dr. Ziem, where he eventually received a complete cure. He was off the charts with cadmium, aluminum, silver, mercury, and a few others. The skin on his entire upper body was slate grey.

Diagnosis was achieved via the Melisa Test.

Dr. Ziem had to design a complete protocol from scratch in order to treat him. This included a strong supplement program, including high doses of Vitamin E and Selenium, as well as healing Calcium Bentonite Clay used internally. No standard chelating agents were used.

The most critical part of Ziem's treatment protocol was very simple: Steam Sauna Therapy. This man literally sweated metals you could wipe off with a towel. This of course would not have been effective without the supplementation.

There is a lot of strong evidence suggesting that clay therapy may be an ideal, if not the ideal, treatment for heavy metal toxicity.

Clay works WITH the human organism, and therefore is dependant on the body's own resources for its action. In severe cases, obviously many of the body's normal functions begin to shut down.

Therefore, I believe we need to consider a few simple principles:

Stimulation and Cleansing.

I recently had a meeting with a brilliant genetic scientist. New research indicates that the immune system makes intelligent choices based on a very wide array of variables. A single effective choice made by the immune system can become an instant habit that is passed, on a cellular level, to the entire immune system. When the body is subjected to substances that induce a toxic response, the immune system literally makes a decision on how this substance is to be dealt with. If the primary objective is achieved, i.e., protection of main circulatory system and organs, then this response will likely be used thereafter. This is not ideal, as the body can choose to try to store these substances if immediate systemic elimination was not possible without deemed risk to the organism."

In conclusion, remember that Calcium Bentonite Clay cannot be used wrong. For a full body detox – get it in you, on you, and all around you in every fashion possible.

DIABETES

Treating diabetes is a fine balancing act. We recommend you first do a complete full body detoxification, monitoring your blood sugar 2-3 times daily. After completing your detox, also insuring your dietary practices are appropriate for your type of diabetes, continue drinking 2-3 ounces of liquid Calcium Bentonite Clay as a daily lifetime practice. We also recommend adding 2-3 ounces of fresh prickly pear pad to your daily diet.

DIAPER RASH

Simply sprinkle the dry powder Calcium Bentonite Clay mixed with arrowroot and cornstarch on your baby's butt as you would powder. If any rash or spots are present, dab on some hydrated Calcium Bentonite Clay. Redness should disappear in 1 day, spots and blisters in 2 days. Continue to use the Calcium Bentonite Clay dry powder mix as your regular baby powder to avoid any rash ever again.

DIARRHEA

Clay is recognized worldwide as a treatment for diarrhea. In China, clay was used for many centuries as a cure for summer diarrhea and cholera. In 1712, Father Deutrecolle, a Jesuit missionary traveling through China, described the clay works there and mentioned that clay was used in treating diarrhea. In fact, as late as 1919, clay proved an invaluable medicine in the cholera epidemic that swept through China.

In times of war, clay has been an outstanding medicine for its healing capabilities. During World War II, French soldiers ate clay to combat dysentery. The use of clay with other medications during the Balkan war of 1910 reduced the mortality from cholera among the soldiers from a high 60 percent to an unbelievably low 3 percent.

Clay has also been used as an adsorptive in the symptomatic treatment of various forms of enteritis, including ulcerative colitis.

Gastrointestinal adsorbents, including clay, are presently recommended for acute diarrhea and bacillary dysentery to adsorb the toxins that produce the diarrhea. Clay has been used in the treatment of abnormal intestinal fermentation to adsorb gases, toxins, and bacteria. In a fluid medium, it carries down large numbers of bacteria and adsorbs the toxins of cholera, typhoid, dysentery, and, apparently, the putrefactive and proteolytic bacteria.

Investigations have indicated that Calcium Bentonite Clay adsorbs viruses, including those of intestinal influenza, in which the diarrhea was controlled in an average of 2.2 days. Calcium Bentonite Clay has antiviral properties.

The clay should be taken frequently: Three ounces of liquid Calcium Bentonite Clay, three times a day, at a minimum. The condition responds better to quick, continued treatment, so repeat the dose often (every two to four hours). When the symptoms disappear, stay on a maintenance dose of one tablespoon a day.

For infants who suffer from diarrhea, add one-fourth to one-half teaspoon of clay to their bottle and shake vigorously. It will mix with the solution, and the infant won't even know it's there.

A study of the therapeutic efficacy of clay for acute diarrhea of diverse causes was reported in the *Medical Annals of the District of Columbia* (Damrau 1961). The causes were virus infection, food allergy, spastic colitis, mucous colitis, and food poisoning. The symptoms evaluated in 35 cases in addition to diarrhea, included abdominal cramps, anorexia, malaise, headache, nausea, and weakness.

The group included 25 women and 10 men. Every effort was made to obtain a homogeneous group of patients so as to eliminate variable from the study.

As a standard treatment, two tablespoons of Calcium Bentonite Clay in distilled water were given three times daily. In cases of food allergy, the dosage was increased to more than six tablespoonfuls daily.

Acute diarrhea was relieved by clay in 34 of the 35 cases (97 percent) in an average time of 3.8 days, and the number of daily bowel movements was reduced to an average of 1.8.

In the 18 cases of diarrhea due to virus infection, the therapeutic response was unusually prompt. In the 8 cases due to food allergy, the diarrhea persisted longer and on many occasions returned if the same allergenic food was eaten again.

The concomitant symptoms of abdominal cramps, anorexia, malaise, headache, nausea, and weakness were also relieved. No side effects attributable to the clay treatment were observed in any case.

Make sure to drink plenty of water with your liquid Calcium Bentonite Clay. Relief should begin by the end of the first day of treatment.

DIVERTICULOSIS

When the colon is not properly emptied, the walls of the intestines form balloons, or diverticula. Soon, undigested food creeps into the pouches and may cause inflammation. The condition, known as diverticulosis, is mainly due to constipation. The clay may be taken frequently to prevent this.

However, if you have already been stricken by the ailment, and you have never taken clay, it is safe to do so. A fast is recommended to speed the healing process. While you fast, take 2-3 ounces of liquid Calcium Bentonite Clay three times per day to adsorb toxins and accelerate the elimination of intestinal waste. Eating clay will also help to form soft stool, which relieves the need to strain. For bulk add psyllum to liquid clay.

DRUG ADDICTION – see Detoxification – Full Body

When changing an addictive lifestyle the process can be eased by first cleansing and detoxing your body.

DRY SKIN – see Skin Health

EARACHE

A three-year-old boy was suffering so much from an infection of the ear that a doctor advised the parents to immediately give antibiotics if they didn't want their son to have complications set in. The father refused to give antibiotics. He called a friend who knew about clay who advised him to apply two to three poultices a day on the back of the ear. After two days the pain was gone. They continued applying the poultices for an extra day or two to make sure that the infection was completely gone.

Use of Calcium Bentonite Clay poultices as described and internal use of liquid Calcium Bentonite Clay offer quick relief of earaches.

Continued use of liquid Calcium Bentonite Clay on a daily basis is a good method of avoiding repeat and chronic earache conditions.

ECZEMA AND PSORIASIS

What are Eczema and Psoriasis?

Eczema is the most common inflammatory disease of the skin and affects many millions of adults and children worldwide. It is estimated that between 10-20% of the world population is affected by this chronic, relapsing, and very itchy rash at some point in their lives. While not uncommon for adults to suffer with eczema, the disease often appears during childhood, or even during infancy. Eczema is a general term for any type of dermatitis or inflammation and itching of the skin; characterized by red, dry scaly skin. Atopic Dermatitis is the most common and severe form of Eczema, so the general term Eczema is often specifically applied to Atopic Dermatitis.

Eczema is caused by an excessive response of the body's immune system to allergens.

Psoriasis is a more rare, yet common skin disease affecting 1% to 2% of the population. The main feature of psoriasis is a red scaly area or patch. The patches appear particularly on the knees, elbows and scalp and sometimes on other parts of the trunk, and legs. Psoriasis can occur at any stage of life although it starts most frequently in young adults. Once thought to be a skin disorder, psoriasis is now understood to be a condition originating in the immune system that can appear in many different forms and can affect any part of the body, including the nails and scalp. It is characterized by skin cells that multiply up to 10 times faster than normal. As underlying cells reach the skin's surface and die, their sheer volume causes raised, red patches covered with white scale.

Although no one single cause for psoriasis has been found, it is known that factors inherited from ones parents are important. An abnormal immune response to some part of the skin is now thought to be central. Involved skin is replaced much more rapidly, and has a more vigorous blood supply. This can lead to redness, scaling, thickening and itching of involved areas of skin.

With both of these diseases, recent scientific study has shown that the body's immune system is the culprit. For some reasons yet unknown, in both these instances, the immune system begins to react abnormally, resulting in these debilitating, heart-breaking conditions. In most cases, these maladies are treated with steroids and other medications with highly questionable side effects. While there is no official cure for either of these diseases, many people have received great relief, and often total removal of symptoms by using Calcium Bentonite Clay.

How Does Calcium Bentonite Clay Help Fight These Diseases?

Calcium Bentonite Clay acts as a magnet and a sponge. It's highly charged negative ions attract all positive charged ions (bacteria, viruses, toxins, etc.) from your body. These substances stick to and are absorbed by the Calcium Bentonite Clay, and are eliminated from your body with the clay. In his book *The Clay Cure*, Ran Knishinsky writes: "When clay is consumed, its vital force is released into the physical body and mingles with the vital energy of the body, creating a stronger, more powerful energy in the host. The natural magnetic action transmits a remarkable power to the organism and helps to re-build vital potential through the liberation of latent energy. When the immune system does not function at its best, the clay stimulates the body's inner resources to awaken the stagnant energy. It supplies the body with the available magnetism to run well. Clay is said to propel the immune system to find a new healthy balance and strengthens the body to a point of higher resistance."

Fight Skin Problems Using the Two-Fisted Approach – 73
Both Externally and Internally

Applications of Calcium Bentonite Clay have been known to be successful in cases of Psoriasis and Eczema. The effective action begins through the electromagnetic process of adsorbing the inflammation in the lesions, along with the deformed cells and dead scales. Pain and itching stop almost instantly following the application of the clay. The clay then assists the body in building new tissue. Smother the affected area with a thick layer of hydrated clay, and then prevent the clay from drying for several hours by wrapping the area with plastic food wrap. Glad Press and Seal works great for this purpose. After several hours, repeat the process with fresh clay and plastic wrap. During the day if the clay wrap is inconvenient just apply the hydrated clay topically in a thin application and let it dry. Re-apply whenever you experience itching.

Combine this program with ingestion of liquefied Calcium Bentonite Clay three times a day. Drink 1 to 2 ounces of liquefied clay three times a day depending on the severity of the condition. Also soak 15-20 minutes at least twice a week in a hot bath into which a cup of powdered clay, or 2-4 cups of liquid Calcium Bentonite Clay has been added. People report that this simultaneous external and internal regimen produces the best results. It may take several months to control or get rid of it depending on how severe it is. Also, It may appear to worsen at first as the dead skin flakes off and circulation is pulled to the area making it look red, but this is temporary.

Most report virtually immediate relief from itching and discomfort. Incorporate Calcium Bentonite Clay as a daily lifetime practice for long-term relief from eczema and psoriasis.

FIBROMYALGIA – see Detoxification – Full Body

FINGERNAIL FUNGUS – see Fungus

FIRE ANT BITES – see Insect Stings and Bites

FLATULENCE – see Gas

FLU – INFLUENZA
Flu is a viral infection and consists of positive charged ions. Calcium Bentonite Clay is extremely effective in removing flu viral molecules from your body. Use as follows:
Days 1-3
Drink 3 ounces liquid Calcium Bentonite Clay three times daily. Take a clay bath daily.
Days 4 – end of symptoms
Same as days 1-3 except reduce liquid clay ingestion to 1 ounce per day.

FOOD POISONING
Clay has proved itself beneficial in the relief of nausea and vomiting. It is an excellent treatment for morning sickness and

food poisoning. In India, clay was found useful in the treatment of acute bacterial food poisonings in the British Army.

In cases of nausea, vomiting, and suspected food poisoning, take one ounce of liquid Calcium Bentonite Clay every two hours as long as needed. Drink plenty of water to help the clay absorb/adsorb the toxins, bacteria, or viruses that are causing the nausea. If the nausea is especially severe, one tablespoon every ten minutes will be helpful. Usually, four tablespoons is enough to halt the symptoms; typically, the nausea will cease within one hour. Thereafter, you can follow up with one dose every four hours until bedtime. This will help to further relieve the gastrointestinal tract and take a heavy burden off the liver.

In addition, the clay is a preferred treatment for any gastrointestinal infections caused by E. coli, Shigella, Salmonella, and Klebsiella, in the same dosages as given above.

FRACTURES – see Broken Bones

FUNGUS
Fungus is normally found under the toenails and fingernails. It is a systemic blood borne pathogen and quite difficult to successfully cure using traditional medicine.

Fortunately, Calcium Bentonite Clay offers a quick, all natural cure for even the worst cases of nail fungus. Use as follows:
Days 1-10
Drink 3 ounces liquid Calcium Bentonite Clay three times a day. Pack hydrated Calcium Bentonite Clay under and on the affected nails and leave on for about 1-2 hours. Repeat this process 3 times daily and leave on overnight.
Days 11-24
Same as days 1-10 except reduce the liquid Calcium Bentonite Clay to 2 ounces twice daily.
Days 25 – until fungus is gone

Reduce liquid Calcium Bentonite Clay to 1 ounce twice daily.

GANGLION CYSTS – see Tumors

GAS
Drink liquid Calcium Bentonite Clay on a daily basis – one ounce twice daily and gas should no longer be a problem.
GINGIVITIS – see Gum Disease

GULF WAR SYNDROME – see Detoxification – Full Body

GUM DISEASE – GINGIVITIS AND PYORRHEA
The clay treatments for gingivitis and pyorrhea are the same (gingivitis will develop into pyorrhea if left untreated). The first line of action involves brushing the teeth daily with Calcium Bentonite Clay. Use clay powder. The clay is absorbent, so it will not be abrasive, and it helps harden the enamel while it aids in gum tissue repair. Furthermore, if used regularly, it helps to prevent gum recession.

Use a toothbrush to apply powdered Calcium Bentonite Clay directly to gums. Do this by loading the toothbrush with powdered clay and gently sweeping it over your gums. Retain it in your mouth (don't rinse your mouth after applying the powdered clay). A practical time to do this would be at bedtime. The powdered clay will slowly dissolve on your gums, under your gums and between your teeth. Make sure to gently press some of the powdered clay below your gums at the gum line. As a preventative measure, brush your teeth daily with powdered clay in the morning and before bed.

HAIR LOSS
Use hydrated Calcium Bentonite Clay daily as you would a cream rinse. Apply thickly to your hair after washing. Leave

on for 5-10 minutes then rinse off. Many have reported new hair growth in as little as 3-4 weeks. Follow shampoo with a cream rinse.

HAY FEVER – see Allergies

HEADACHES – MIGRAINES

Because headaches are rooted in so many causes, the treatment approach must be host centered and broad spectrum. And if the cause of the headaches is due in part to chemical sensitivities, food allergies, or circulation of toxins in the body, the Calcium Bentonite Clay will enable the body to detoxify more efficiently and utilize nutrients more effectively.

The treatment is the same whether the headache/migraine is due to muscle tension, chemical imbalance, analgesic rebound or any of 100 other causations for the problem.

Upon onset of the headache, drink 3 ounces liquid Calcium Bentonite Clay. Repeat 3 times daily.

Soak a washcloth in cool liquid Calcium Bentonite Clay and place across the nape of the neck for about 30 minutes. Rinse and resoak the washcloth with liquid Calcium Bentonite Clay and place on the forehead for about 30 minutes. Repeat this process as often as you like until the pain dissipates.

If headaches are frequent and reoccurring, do a full body detox as a treatment and continue drinking 1 ounce of liquid Calcium Bentonite Clay twice daily as a life practice.

HEART HEALTH

According to Michael Abehsara, author of *The Healing Clay*, Calcium Bentonite Clay is rich in diastases (enzymes), which account for its ability to fix free oxygen and purify and enrich the blood. Free radicals are atoms whose electrons have been stripped; while a certain number of them are necessary to stave off invading bacteria, too many can attack the body, causing cellular breakdown. Clay contributes to an improved blood supply.

High levels of blood risk factors, such as too many free radicals, help to explain the breakdown of the cardiovascular system in the form of strokes or heart attacks. If the body continues to pump dirty blood to the heart, heart disease is sure to follow. The vessel walls are eventually weakened by weak blood, which cannot carry the nutrients needed for blood vessel reinforcement. Clay's cleansing action on the stomach, small intestine, and colon may prevent this.

To help prevent heart disease, or as part of a "healthy heart" plan following heart surgery or a heart attack, we recommend the following.

Days 1-14

Drink 2 ounces liquid Calcium Bentonite Clay three times daily. Take a clay bath in the morning.

Days 15-45

Drink 1 ounce liquid Calcium Bentonite Clay three times daily. Take 3 clay baths weekly.

As a lifestyle practice, drink 1-2 ounces liquid Calcium Bentonite Clay daily and take a weekly clay bath.

HEMORRHOIDS

Hemorrhoids are varicose veins in the anus and colon, possibly resulting from pushing and straining when going to the restroom. They can become quite painful.

Use as follows:

Days 1-7

Drink 2 ounces liquid, three times daily. Insert 1 Calcium Bentonite Clay suppository in the morning and evening. Take a daily clay bath.

Days 8-21

Drink 1 ounce liquid Calcium Bentonite Clay three times daily. Insert one suppository in the morning. Take 3 clay baths per week.

As a daily practice drink 1 ounce liquid Calcium Bentonite Clay and take a weekly clay bath.

HEPATITIS

For hepatitis begin with a full body detoxification. Hepatitis directly affects the liver but is systemic in nature. After a detoxification has been completed begin the following treatment regimen.

Drink 3 ounces liquid Calcium Bentonite Clay three times daily. Take a clay bath once daily. Apply a 1" thick clay poultice, approximately 12" in diameter to your liver area, twice daily, for 30 minutes.

After 2 weeks of the above treatment, reduce the liquid Calcium Bentonite Clay to 2 ounces in the morning and in the evening.

After 1 month of treatment reduce the liquid Calcium Bentonite Clay to 1 ounce twice daily. Reduce the clay baths to 3 per week. Reduce the poultice to 1 per day.

79

You should well be on your way to a full recovery.

HERPES – COLD SORES

Herpes is a sexually transmitted viral with outbreaks on the lips and genitals. The outbreaks are intermittent and appear as fluid filled blisters. This is a highly contagious viral when outbreaks are present.

As you know, all virals are of a positive charged ionic molecule. Calcium Bentonite Clay's negatively charged properties will remove this viral from your body through absorption and adsorption.

As herpes simplex virus is blood borne and systemic, you should begin your Calcium Bentonite Clay treatment with a full body detoxification regimen – see Detoxification – Full Body.

Follow that process with daily ingestion of 2 ounces liquid Calcium Bentonite Clay and 3 weekly clay baths. Continue until your body shows no remaining traces of the virus.

HIVES

Hives are a skin rash that is typically due to an allergic reaction. Please see "Allergies" for treatment in this case. In addition, topical applications of hydrated Calcium Bentonite Clay can be used on specific outbreak areas.

INDIGESTION

Indigestion is one of the easiest maladies to cure using Calcium Bentonite Clay. Oftentimes complete relief comes in 10-15 seconds after ingestion!

Treat as follows:

Drink 2 ounces liquid Calcium Bentonite Clay three times daily and at any time indigestion occurs. Continue this daily practice for 2-3 days or until full relief is present. As a daily maintenance dose, drink 1 ounce liquid Calcium Bentonite Clay twice daily and at any time any sign of indigestion appears.

INFECTIONS – STAPH, GANGRENE, ETC.

Most infections are systemic, blood borne with localized sores on the skin. Treatment of an infection is both full body and localized on the open wounds or skin sores.

Days 1-4

Drink 3 ounces liquid Calcium Bentonite Clay three times daily. Take a clay bath daily. Cover the open wound or skin sore with thick hydrated Calcium Bentonite Clay. Cover with plastic wrap. Leave on for 2-3 hours and do not allow the Calcium Bentonite Clay to dry. You may also apply a large clay poultice to the outbreak area. Repeat the clay covering of the wound 3 times daily.

Days 5-10

Reduce liquid clay to 2 ounces twice daily. Stay with the same three applications daily of hydrated Calcium Bentonite Clay or poultices until would is closed.

Days 11 on

Continue to drink 1 ounce of Calcium Bentonite Clay twice daily until infection is completely gone from your body. Take clay baths and cover the outbreak area with clay as desired until infection is completely gone.

IMMUNO DEFICIENCY – see AIDS

Although AIDS is quite different from a traditional immuno deficiency, the treatment is the same.

INSECT STINGS & BITES

Treatment for any type of insect sting or bite is the same, whether it is from a wasp, mosquito, bee or any other insect.

Immediately dab on a good finger full of hydrated Calcium Bentonite Clay. Cover the bite area and about another 1" all around the bite area. Leave on to dry or cover with plastic wrap.

Repeat this process 3-10 times until all pain, swelling, redness, etc., has passed.

Pain normally begins to leave in as little as 30 seconds to 1 minute. Complete relief usually occurs in 3-5 applications over a few hours.

IRRITABLE BOWEL SYNDROME - IBS

This ailment is characterized by alternating conditions of diarrhea and constipation with gas, pain, and emotional ups and downs. Because the cause of irritable bowel syndrome is unknown, treating the condition with drugs can be dangerous. Even naturopathic doctors have a difficult time in controlling, managing, and curing the disease.

Clay is an excellent choice for this very real ailment. Begin by doing an internal and colon cleanse. Please see that section and treat in the appropriate fashion.

Once relief is experienced from the cleanse, maintain daily ingestion of liquid Calcium Bentonite Clay. Drink 1-2 ounces liquid Calcium Bentonite Clay daily and the problem should not reoccur.

ITCHY SKIN – see Hives

KIDNEY STONES

Kidney stones can effectively be treated using the following treatment plan. Although complete removal of the stones may take 1-3 months. Treat as follows:

Days 1-7

Drink 3 ounces liquid Calcium Bentonite Clay three times daily. Take a clay bath daily. Apply a ½" thick by 12" in diameter clay poultice over each kidney for about 30 minutes. Repeat this 3 times daily.

Days 8-30

Drink 2 ounces liquid Calcium Bentonite Clay 3 times daily. Take 4-5 clay baths weekly. Apply clay poultices described above twice daily.

Days 31-60

Drink 1 ounce liquid Calcium Bentonite Clay 3 times daily. Take 2-3 clay baths weekly. Apply clay poultices described above once daily.

Days 61-on

Until all traces of kidney stones are gone drink 1 ounce of liquid Calcium Bentonite Clay twice daily. Take 1-2 clay baths weekly. Apply poultices as described above once daily.

LACTATION – see Pregnancy

LEAKY GUT SYNDROME

Please see the treatment regimen for Irritable Bowel Syndrome – IBS. Although the locations along the digestive path where these two ailments occur are different, the treatment plan is the same.

LIPOFUSCIN ABNORMALITIES

Calcium Bentonite Clay works for all types of skin coloration abnormalities. Skin coloration abnormalities are caused by either an abnormal buildup or absence of pigment – lipofuscin. Calcium Bentonite Clay creates a balance of pigment in any affected area. It will reduce age spots (liver spots) completely in about 4 weeks with daily applications. Birthmarks are transformed, as are other forms of skin discoloration with applications of Calcium Bentonite Clay as follows:

Drink 2 ounces of liquid Calcium Bentonite Clay daily. Apply hydrated Calcium Bentonite Clay in a relatively thick coating to the discolored area. Allow to dry and leave on for 45-60 minutes. Wash and reapply 3-4 times daily. Leave the last application on overnight and wash off in the morning.

Continue this treatment until skin has changed to the desired level of color.

LIVER CLEANSE

The liver is frequently referred to as the body's detoxification pilot. It breaks down poisons or transforms them into less harmful compounds. The poisons include toxins found in food (nitrates, monosodium glutamate, and herbicides), toxins produced by the body (ketones, indoles, phenols, and aldehydes), as well as toxins in the environment. In addition, the liver performs a long list of other functions, including the manufacture of bile salts, the activation of vitamin D, and storage of glycogen, vitamin A, copper, and iron. The liver, without a doubt, is absolutely vital to one's health.

Calcium Bentonite Clay can be an invaluable aid to a poorly functioning liver. It works indirectly on the organ, as follows. After you eat, the absorption of nutrients takes place throughout the length of the small intestine and the large intestine. From here they are transported in the bloodstream to the liver by way of the hepatic portal system (the flow of blood from the digestive organs to the liver). After their passage through the liver, they move through the heart and then enter general circulation.

If the bowels are not working right, waste matter will be continually reabsorbed into the blood stream and carried to the liver. As a result, the liver is forced into doing extra work that might not be needed if the bowels were in good working condition. This places an unnecessary burden on the liver and the rest of the body. Eating clay will have a positive effect on the liver by facilitating the cleansing of the gastrointestinal tract. Through adsorption and absorption, many of the toxins

will exit directly through the colon and bypass the liver and general circulation. Further, because the Kupffer cells of the liver, which respond to the chemical balance of the colon, govern immune function, intestinal health is integral to quality liver function. Although clay does not work directly on the organ, its actions are soon felt there.

As the treatment is internal and Detox related, follow the treatment protocol outlined in the full body Detoxification section.

LYMPHATITIS – LYMPH GLANDS
Lymphatitis is treated both internally and topically. Begin by completing a full body detox and internal cleanse (see those ailment sections).

Since Lymph is present throughout our body a full system cleanse is the requisite first step. In addition add hot clay baths 2 times a week.

Continue drinking 2 ounces liquid Calcium Bentonite Clay twice daily until the lymph glands and full system is back to health.

If there is any swelling or tenderness in any specific glands, such as under arms, neck, etc., apply a poultice directly to the affected glands. Leave on for 30 minutes and repeat twice daily. Continue until system is again in balance.

MENSTRUAL CRAMPS – see Premenstrual Syndrome (PMS)

MERCURY TOXICITY – AMALGAM FILLINGS

Mercury toxicity can be deadly as can poisoning from many other common metals such as lead and cadmium. In the past few years we have learned of the mercury poisoning from old amalgam fillings.

No matter what type of metal poisoning or from what source the toxicity is derived, the treatment is the same. Please see Detoxification – Full Body for the treatment regimen. Take regular pH and metal level tests as your benchmarks for progress and to know when all toxic metals have been removed from your body.

MIGRAINES – see Headaches

MOLES – see Warts

MOSQUITO BITES – see Insect Bites

MOUTH ULCERS

Mouth ulcers are easily treated with Calcium Bentonite Clay. Since the inside of our mouths are wet, you can dab on, or sprinkle on, some dry powder Calcium Bentonite Clay, allowing it to stick to the ulcerated area. You may also apply a thick dab of hydrated Calcium Bentonite Clay to the ulcer.

Allow the Calcium Bentonite Clay to remain in place as long as possible. As it dissolves or is washed away, simply swallow and reapply throughout the day.

MUMPS

This inflammation of the salivary and parotid glands may affect the testicles, ovaries, mammary glands, pancreas, and thyroid. Treat with liquid Calcium Bentonite Clay and poultices as follows:

Drink 2 ounces liquid Calcium Bentonite Clay twice daily during the duration of the inflammation. Also, place poultices over the inflamed areas for about 30 minutes 3 times daily.

This should cut the normal healing time in half and better protect other organs as well.

MUSCLE SORENESS – CRAMPS

Muscle soreness, as well as problems with muscle cramping are easily remedied with Calcium Bentonite Clay.

As a first course of action take a hot Calcium Bentonite Clay bath. Relief should occur in less than 30 minutes. Repeat this Calcium Bentonite Clay bath for several days.

You may also want to treat specific areas of soreness or cramping with applications of hydrated Calcium Bentonite Clay. Simply apply the Calcium Bentonite Clay to the entire affected area rather thickly and cover with plastic wrap. Leave on for 1-2 hours then wash off. You may repeat this process 3 times daily if necessary.

Drink 2ounces liquid Calcium Bentonite Clay twice daily during the period in which you are experiencing muscle cramps or soreness.

NAUSEA AND VOMITING

Although nausea and vomiting are not necessarily the result of food poisoning, the treatment with Calcium Bentonite

Clay is the same. Please see Food Poisoning for treatment of nausea or vomiting due to any factors.

NUCLEAR RADIATION DETOXIFICATION

The Russians used Calcium Bentonite Clay to clean up after Chernobyl. The U.S. government uses Calcium Bentonite Clay as a protectant to line the walls of its nuclear fallout shelters. There is nothing more effective at removing nuclear radiation from your body than Calcium Bentonite Clay. After Chernobyl the Russian soldiers passed out chocolate bars made with Bentonite to children to get clay in them.

Please see "Detoxification – Full Body" for treatment protocol.

OILY SKIN – see Skin Health

PARASITES

The vast majority of Americans in today's society have par- asites. I'm talking about hookworms, pinworms, roundworms, tapeworms, and countless other nasty creatures. Theresa Schumacher, co-author of *Cleansing the Body and the Colon for a Happier and Healthier You*, estimates there are "about 300 different types of parasites thriving in America today." In recent medical studies, it has been estimated that 85% of the North American adult population has at least one form of parasite living in their bodies. Some authorities feel that this figure may be as high as 95%.

Dr. Peter Wina, Chief of the Patho-Biology in the Walter Reed Army Institute of Research, states, "We have a tremendous parasite problem right here in the U.S. It is just not being addressed."

Dr. Frank Nova, Chief of the Laboratory for Parasitic Diseases of the National Institute of Health, says, "In terms of numbers there are more parasitic infections acquired in this country than in Africa."

This is something we must take very seriously. The combination of environmental toxins, an unhealthy diet and parasites poses a grave danger to humans. "In fact, parasites have killed more humans than all the wars in history," reported *National Geographic* in its award-winning documentary, *The Body Snatchers*.

The immediate question that comes to mind when people are informed of this situation is: How can a parasite possibly live in my body and I don't even know it is there? The answer to this is simple. The purpose of a parasite is to not make itself known. A smart parasite lives without being detected because if it is detected, of course, something is going to be done to eradicate it. If you think parasites are stupid, think again. They are highly intelligent organisms. Not intelligent in the same way humans are, but they are intelligent in their ability to survive and reproduce, which is of course, the purpose of any organism on this planet.

Dr. Ross Andersen, N.D. puts it this way, "Other prominent physicians agree with me; that in human history, the parasite challenge is likely the most unrecognized of all endemic problems. Because they cannot be seen and rarely present immediate symptoms, they remain invisible as a cause or contributing factor to what can be a serious disorder."

We don't know why every generation prior to modern times made de-worming a regular part of their lives, but our generation chooses to ignore this basic practice. It is recognized that people in third world countries have parasites. It is also recognized that most of the animals we eat, and pets who live in our homes have an innumerable number of parasites and worms, but for whatever reason we seem to dismiss the notion that we as a modern society might also have foreign entities living within us as well. For whatever reason the medical profession chooses to try to downplay this fact, but the public is rapidly becoming more and more aware of this knowledge.

Parasites live everywhere and are commonly transmitted to humans in diverse ways, such as insect bites, walking barefoot, human contact, animal contact, drinking water, eating undercooked meats and fish, and numerous other ways. Government inspectors do not inspect most of the animals that go through the slaughterhouse. What about salads, or even raw fruits and vegetables? Eating raw foods always increases the risk of parasites. According to the Center of Disease Control (CDC), illnesses linked with fruits and vegetables are on the rise. One reason could be the increased demand for fresh produce. We now import 30 billion tons of food a year. Some of the produce comes from developing nations where sanitation facilities are less advanced or they commonly practice the use of human feces as fertilizer (night soil). The further products travel, the more likely they will pick up illness-causing microbes. It also increases the chance of being contaminated by infected food handlers. Food handlers have been in the news lately because of their role in the spread of parasites. Some people who prepare food, as well as the general population do not wash their hands after going to the bathroom. When you consider that many of the parasites are spread by fecal-oral contact, this lack of personal hygiene may be one of the greatest factors in the spread of parasites. Consider everything that you touch that is handled by others; money, shopping carts, door handles, menus, saltshakers, and everything else — the possibilities for contamination are enormous.

Why Are So Many of Us Infested with Parasites?

The problem lies within our digestive system. Theresa Schumacher's book lists several types of parasites and a variety of ways in which they are caught. As for parasites in food, Schumacher notes the parasite incubation period is 36 hours. She says once we have eaten a meal we should be able to eliminate the waste from that food within 16 to 24 hours. But, she notes, "It is startling to learn that the average elimination time in America today is 96 hours."

If waste is not eliminated within 24 hours, it begins a toxic buildup that provides a breeding ground for parasitic infection. She writes that a clogged intestine with putrid fecal matter and plenty of sugar provides the ideal environment for parasites to thrive. It is now common knowledge that the average American adult has between 10-20 pounds of putrefying waste matter lodged in their intestines.

This waste material is home to, in the words of *National Geographic*, "a sinister world of monstrous creatures that feed on living flesh: parasites." *Discover* magazine published a feature article in its August 2000 issue:

"Every living thing has at least one parasite that lives inside or on it, and many, including humans, have far more. Scientists are only just beginning to discover exactly how powerful these hidden inhabitants can be, but their research is pointing to a remarkable possibility: Parasites may rule the world. The notion that tiny creatures we've largely taken for granted are such a dominant force is immensely disturbing. We are collections of cells that work together, kept harmonized by chemical signals. If an organism can control those signals — an organism like a parasite — then it can control us. And therein lies the peculiar and precise horror of parasites."

Infestations may be severe or mild and can be life threatening, especially for children. A common side affect is the poor absorption of critical nutrients for growth potentially leading to anemia, growth problems, and a weakened immune function creating susceptibility for disease. According to numerous books, parasites are commonly found in people with AIDS, chronic fatigue syndrome, candidiasis, and many other disorders. Symptoms may include abdominal pains, diarrhea, anemia, cardiac insufficiency, nausea, perianal & perineal pruritis, dysentery, amebic hepatitis, weight loss, intestinal toxemia, colic and cirrhosis.

Schumacher, states a clogged-up colon and its parasitic infection is often the undiagnosed root of many physical problems. But, Schumacher writes, the medical profession "does not even agree with the notion of filthy and impacted colons contributing to much American ill health. This may be because there are no patented drugs for quick relief of impacted colons. The only way to cleanse intestines is with natural ingredients, and via a persistent personal hygiene program."

In his book, *The Clay Cure*, Ran Knishinsky writes:

"While many herbs and homeopathic remedies are suggested for this condition, I believe Calcium Bentonite Clay offers the finest treatments for all types of parasites. First, its use will stimulate the gall bladder to increase the flow of bile according to Raymond Dextreit, a French naturopath. He writes that no parasite can live too long under any bilious condition.

Second, considerable research has shed light on the connection between clay eating and parasites. The *American Journal of Clinical Nutrition* mentioned this in a recent article: "Geophagy can be a source of nutrients. Its primary way of enhancing nutritional status appears to be, however, to counter dietary toxins and, secondarily, the effects of gastrointestinal parasites" (Johns and Duquette 1991). Further, numerous citations in a host of other journals collaborate this fact: throughout the globe, people eat clay in response to parasites.

Third, worms are themselves clay-eaters and are attracted to clay. As a result, when the clay is eliminated from the body, so are the worms."

According to Joseph Sterling, editor of the health newsletter *Secrets of Robust Health*, "Humans can play host to over 100 different kinds of parasites, ranging from microscopic to several feet long tapeworms. Contrary to popular belief, parasites are not restricted to our colon alone, but can be found in other parts of the body; the lungs, the liver, in the muscles and joints, in the esophagus, the brain, the blood, the skin and even in the eyes."

In his article for the monthly newsletter, Joseph Sterling lists the following as common symptoms of parasitic infection:
Constipation
Gas and bloating
Diarrhea
Pains or aches in the back, joints or muscles
Irritable bowel syndrome
Allergies
Eating more than normal but still being hungry
Itchy ears, nose or anus
Unpleasant sensations in the stomach
Nervousness or grumpiness
Chronic fatigue, lethargy or apathy
Various skin problems
Problems sleeping
Nutritional deficiencies or anemia
Immune system problems
Tooth grinding or clenching
Excess weight
Forgetfulness
Blurry vision

These symptoms could have a variety of other causes, but why take the chance when the remedy is at hand? As Dr. Bernard Jensen and countless others have recommended for years, use Calcium Bentonite Clay to detoxify your body and rid it of parasites.

Please see Detoxification – Full Body, for treatment regime.

PH BALANCE

Calcium Bentonite Clay is the great pH balancer! A healthy body maintains about a 7.4 pH. In an acidic environment (less than 7.4) disease flourishes.

Calcium Bentonite Clay has a pH as high as 9.7. To change the pH of your body from acid to alkaline, simply get the clay in you and on you. Calcium Bentonite Clay has a favorable effect on every function of your body.

Drink 1-2 ounces of Calcium Bentonite Clay daily. Take 2-3 clay baths weekly. Do one full body wrap weekly.

Test your pH with inexpensive, easy to use, saliva test strips. Adjust the amount of Calcium Bentonite Clay needed to fine-tune your body's pH level.

PIMPLES – see Acne

PINK EYE
Treat as follows:

Take a 2" by 2" telfa pad and open one side with scissors. Open the pad and fill with hydrated Calcium Bentonite Clay. Close the "Clay Pad" and lay over the affected eye for 30-45 minutes. Repeat 3-4 times per day. Also drink 2 ounces liquid Calcium Bentonite Clay daily until ailment is gone.

POISON
The nutritionist Linda Clark mentions in her recent book, *The Best of Linda Clark*, that a European doctor, Meyer-Camberg, recommends clay for neutralizing poisons. According to Dr. Meyer-Camberg, clay can take care of any bad poisoning, even arsenic!

The *American Journal of Medicine* published a study conducted with Paraquat, a widely used herbicide, in an effort to understand how medicinal therapy can help avoid a fatal outcome. Doctors fed lethal doses of the herbicide to rats and recorded the effects. They noted than an excess of the poison caused respiratory failure, liver damage, and kidney failure, which soon led to death.

Several adsorbents were shown to be effective in counteracting the effects of the poison before the poison was ingested.

Only one adsorbent proved successful in counteracting the toxic effects of the poison *after* it was ingested: Calcium Bentonite Clay.

In this experimental situation, clay was given in repeated doses rather than single doses. The effectiveness of repeated doses is apparently due to its ability to prevent the gastrointestinal absorption of Paraquat, which can continue up to 30 hours after ingesting in rats. Surprisingly, even when the treatment was delayed for 10 hours after the oral administration of Paraquat, the therapy was successful. The rats did not die and toxic damage was minimal.

The authors of the report went on to say that since urinary Paraquat levels have been detected for as long as 31 days after ingestion, continued efforts, as well as early efforts to eliminate absorbed Paraquat might be important. Therefore, continual use of the clay is advisable because of its ongoing adsorptive properties.

Although the use of Calcium Bentonite Clay as an antidote to poisons has been known for centuries, and the scientific reasons for its success have been known for decades, it is strange that, in a world where heavy metal solutions, alkaloids, cationic pesticides and detergents could be accidentally ingested, Calcium Bentonite Clay is not yet included in Red Cross or First Aid Boxes in factories, homes and chemical laboratories.

If poisoned, immediately begin drinking 2 ounces of liquid Calcium Bentonite Clay every hour for 6-10 hours. Phone the poison control center to learn if it's better to induce vomiting as well or to allow it to pass through your system. Immediate attention is required in any case.

Continue with the liquid clay for the next few days at the rate of 2 ounces Calcium Bentonite Clay twice daily.

POISON IVY OR OAK
Although poison ivy and poison oak inflammations are quite different in causation from hives, the treatment is the

same. Please see the treatment protocol for hives when treating these ailments.

PREGNANCY

A pilgrim from El Salvador and her grown-up daughter browsing among the market stalls around the basilica enthusiastically claimed that they ate the holy tables (clay), and when asked, "Do they do you any good?" the woman's sparkling eyes and instant response was: "Of course they do: I have eight children!" -John M. Hunter and Oscar H. Horst, *National Geographic Research*

A mother-to-be sometimes has strange cravings. For no apparent reason, her body suddenly feels starved for certain inedible substances such as charcoal, chalk or plain dirt. She will go out of her way to eat them, sneaking into the backyard to scoop up a tiny bit of mud in her hand to suck on, or running into the front yard to peel park off a tree and chew it as if it were a piece of gum. If you ask her why she does this, she may shrug or say, "I don't know, no special reason," or she might say, "I just like it."

Even though these pregnant earth-eaters may not be able to explain their reasons, I believe their actions hold a purpose. Intuitively, the body makes its needs known through physical cravings. When they are responded to, our bodies are "fulfilled" and we are compensated with health. In this case, the mother and her newborn are rewarded.

Well, here's good news for those mothers who run to the backyard to grab a handful of dirt but don't know why: There is a type of dirt they can safely eat – clay. Calcium Bentonite Clay eating is most common during pregnancy, and it is said to be the most favorable practice a mother can undertake for herself and her unborn child.

The following reports explain the many uses of clay by pregnant women everywhere.

Before Pregnancy

Eaten by women who want to bear children. The clay is supposed to have an effect during normal menstruation, before conception has occurred. It is taken as a means of encouraging future pregnancy.

Recommended for women who are sterile.

Good for cleaning the body, creating a better environment to house an infant.

During Pregnancy

It is believed that the unborn infant benefits from it.

Promotes healthy digestion.

Prevents and/or counteracts morning sickness.

Among the women in one culture, it is thought the fetus will be bigger if the mother eats clay.

Helps with minor discomforts.

Has mineral rich nutrient contents.

Gives the fetus "good bones and teeth."

Protects against any unfortunate mishap during pregnancy.

Calcium Bentonite Clay will calm stomach acidity.

Calcium Bentonite Clay adsorbs metabolic toxins such as steroidal metabolites associated with pregnancy.

Delivery

The clay is placed on the tongue of a woman in the belief it facilitates delivery and expulsion of the afterbirth.

The fetus rises in the womb, making delivery easier.

Calcium Bentonite Clay eases labor pains, accelerates the delivery, and strengthens the expectant mother.

Breastfeeding

Women rub their breasts with a paste made from clay to stimulate the secretion of milk.

Taken internally, it is considered good for lactation.

Before I go any further, you may already be wondering, "That's fine that so many women take clay. But how do I know it is really safe for me and my child?"

Yes, eating clay is a safe and suitable practice that can be maintained during pregnancy. But, as I have emphasized throughout the book, it is important to find the *right* clay. Not all clays are good for eating. You want a clean, natural, Calcium Bentonite Clay. Throughout pregnancy, drink 1 ounce liquid Calcium Bentonite Clay daily and take a weekly clay bath.

PREMENSTRUAL SYNDROME – PMS

Eating clay is therapeutic in cases of menstrual cramps. By drawing the metabolic waste products and improving intestinal health, clay helps prevent cramps and lessens the related symptoms (headaches, bloating, irritability). Many naturopaths agree that menstrual cramps are not only a hormonal matter, but are partly due to constipation. One ounce of liquid Calcium Bentonite Clay taken twice per day will be helpful.

If major troubles occur – if the menstruation is very abundant, insufficient, too painful, or accompanied by several clots or mucosities, apply a clay poultice on the lower abdomen every night before going to bed, which should be kept on overnight unless it causes discomfort. For minor troubles it is sometimes sufficient to apply these poultices for 10 days preceding menstruation. Interrupt the application during the menstrual period, after that, resume applying them.

The applications can be continued even if the menstruation takes the form of hemorrhage; *be sure to slightly warm up the poultices in order not to create a congestive state.*

For long-term sufferers of the emotional roller coaster, which oftentimes precedes a menstrual cycle, we recommend drinking liquid Calcium Bentonite Clay as a daily lifestyle practice.

When tackling the symptoms of PMS, for the first 7 days, drink 2 ounces liquid Calcium Bentonite Clay twice daily. Following that, drink 1 ounce liquid Calcium Bentonite Clay as a lifetime practice.

PROSTATE HEALTH

The prostate is located between the rectum and the neck of the bladder. Because of its location, its health can be directly influenced by the condition of the bowels. An impacted colon will undoubtedly affect the health of the prostate. Therefore, a cleansing program is the first thing to implement in any prostate rebuilding program.

Calcium Bentonite Clay will help to prevent the accumulation of waste matter and feces that can clog up the rectum. This could help to diminish the possibility of any future prostate problems, or remedy a current one.

If you suffer from an enlarged prostate, urine leakage or erectile dysfunction we recommend the following treatment.

Days 1-7

Drink 2 ounces liquid Calcium Bentonite Clay twice daily. Use one Calcium Bentonite Clay suppository daily. Take one clay bath daily.

Day 8 – on

Drink 1 ounce liquid Calcium Bentonite Clay daily. Take one clay bath weekly.

PSORIASES – see Eczema

PYORRHEA – see Gum Disease

RADIATION EXPOSURE

It seems that clay has, among other properties, the ability to either stimulate a deficiency or absorb an excess of the radioactivity in the body on which it is applied. On an organism that has suffered and still retains the radiations of radium (or any other intensive radioactive source), the radioactivity is first enhanced and then absorbed. Clay could, in this way, ensure the protection of organisms over-exposed to atomic radiations.

This radioactive effect has been researched: Today, when everyone is forcibly submitted to many artificially provoked radioactive aggressions, such as dust in the atmosphere from bomb testing, everything increasing this danger should be avoided. Experiments made with the Geiger counter have demonstrated that dry clay absorbs a very important part of this surrounding radioactivity.

In the event of a dirty bomb, Living clay can be your best friend. If you are exposed to excess radiation, lather up with hydrated clay from head to toe. Scrub the body and allow the clay to remain on for 10-15 minutes. Wash off thoroughly. Add a cup of powdered clay to your washing machine then wash your clothes again with soap.

Take clay baths with 2- 4 cups of powdered clay added to hot bath water and soak the entire body for 15-20 minutes. Do this daily as long as the danger of radiation is still in the atmosphere.

Drink liquid clay—4 ounces three times a day—and increase in the event of nausea and signs of radiation sickness. If in doubt take more.

RADIATION THERAPY DETOXIFICATION – see Detoxification – Full Body

RINGWORM – see Parasites

ROSACEA
Rosacea is the flushing (reddening) of the skin, usually localized in the face and neck area.

Drink 1-2 ounces of Calcium Bentonite Clay liquid daily. Take 1-2 clay baths weekly.

Over a 4-8 week period you will notice a greatly reduced number of outbreaks. Clay facials every other day.

SCALD – see Burns

SCAR REMOVAL – STRETCH MARKS

Scar removal, both the knotting, keloid effect, as well as the discoloration can be remedied in a period of 1-4 months. Stretch marks, such as those occurring as a result of pregnancy are a bit more difficult an issue.

Stretch marks are literally a separation, a tearing of the outermost layer of your skin, and it is impossible to put those tears back together again. What Calcium Bentonite Clay will do, over a period of several months, is tighten the 3 under layers of skin, oftentimes dramatically, in turn pulling the skin nearer together and tighter than had been the case before. And over a period of 6-12 months the Calcium Bentonite Clay will in fact partially repair and mend the tears of the outer layer of skin. You will experience a noticeable, visually aesthetic improvement.

Scar treatment is quite successful and oftentimes quite dramatic. Treat as follows:

Days 1-15

Drink 2 ounces liquid Calcium Bentonite Clay twice daily. Soak the scar in a clay liquid bath for 30-45 minutes daily. Apply hydrated Calcium Bentonite Clay to the scar and surrounding area. Cover with plastic and leave on for 1 hour. Repeat 3 times daily. Leave the last daily application on overnight.

Days 16 – end of treatment

Drink 1 ounce Calcium Bentonite Clay once daily. Apply hydrated Calcium Bentonite Clay to the scar and surrounding area twice daily, morning and evening. Leave the evening application on overnight.

SCRATCHES – see Abrasions

SEXUALLY TRANSMITTED DISEASES – STD's

STD's are usually systemic, blood borne, and require a full body detoxification at the outset. Please read and treat yourself as per the protocol outlined in that section.

Follow the detox with topical treatments to any affected outbreak areas. Coat liberally with hydrated Calcium Bentonite Clay the entire affected area and 2-3 inches of the surrounding area. Leave on until dry. Reapply 3 times daily.

Drink 2 ounces liquid Calcium Bentonite Clay daily until all symptoms disappear.

SHINGLES – see Eczema
While eczema and shingles are very different when comparing causations, the treatments are exactly the same.

SINUSITIS
If you suffer from sinusitis, dissolve powder Calcium Bentonite Clay in a bowl of steaming water (use about three tablespoons per quart of water). Place a towel over your head (and over the bowl of steaming water and clay mixture) and inhale the steam deeply through your nose. After this, make a compress by soaking a cloth in a mixture of clay and hot water. Lie down and cover your face with the hot, wet compress. Repeat.

SKIN CANCER LESIONS – see Cancer

SKIN HEALTH
The skin is the largest organ and a means of eliminating waste; each day waste passes through the pores of the skin.

Everything that affects the body in turn affects the skin. When the body is full of toxic wastes and cannot eliminate them properly, various skin ailments may result. The only effective way to get rid of these conditions is by cleansing the body inside and out.

I get people all the time complaining about "skin cures" making conditions worse. Most skin conditions are first liver conditions. I pull out a simple pH strip, and measure their saliva. If the saliva pH is below 6.5, I explain that as long as the body needs to dump excessive waste through the skin, then their skin problem will continue.

I explain that Calcium Bentonite Clay can help alleviate this condition. Remember, what we're dealing with is organ failure.

The acids deposited in the skin coupled with the disturbance in the moisture balance of the skin simply create a nice breeding ground for further infection.

Skin conditions that are the result of other problems, such as the condition of the skin itself (oily skin, etc.), respond extremely quickly to Calcium Bentonite Clay.

Treatment is both internal and external and should be used at your own discretion and choice of modality based on your own progress.

Drink 1-2 ounces liquid Calcium Bentonite Clay daily. Take a clay bath 1-2 times weekly. Do a full body wrap and leave on for 20 minutes, 3 times weekly.

Note your skin change daily and take regular pH saliva tests to monitor your progress.

SNAKE BITES

Venomous snakebites require emergency measures and immediate treatment. If a hospital is nearby or if you have access to ambulance assistance, by all means use these life saving emergency services.

After medical treatment also apply a 1" thick poultice, 6" in diameter to the affected area. Leave on for 15 minutes and apply a new poultice. Repeat this process 6-8 times as often as needed. It will help reduce swelling as well as help pull out the venom. In addition drink 2 ounces of liquid Calcium Bentonite 3 times a day as needed.

SORE THROAT

Treat a sore throat in 3 ways. First, gargle with liquid clay for 3-5 minutes. Secondly, soak a washcloth in warm liquid

Calcium Bentonite Clay and lay it across your throat for about 30 minutes.

And third, apply a thin coat of hydrated Calcium Bentonite Clay to your entire throat and neck area. Leave on for an hour or so. Reapply in the evening and leave on overnight.

Calcium Bentonite Clay will cut your healing time in half.

SPIDER BITES

Spider bites fall into one of 2 categories – emergency, which are possibly life threatening, such as a Brown Recluse bite - and nuisance bites, the ones that may raise a small bump and itch a little.

If bitten by a known venomous spider, seek immediate emergency treatment if you have access to a hospital, or if an ambulance can reach your location quickly.

To treat with Calcium Bentonite Clay, immediately drink 6 ounces liquid Calcium Bentonite Clay and apply a thick Calcium Bentonite Clay poultice to the bite and the surrounding area. Change the poultice every 15-20 minutes and continue for 2-4 hours of repeated treatments. Finally apply a heavy coat of hydrated Calcium Bentonite Clay, cover with plastic wrap and leave on overnight.

For nuisance spider bites, apply a coating of hydrated Calcium Bentonite Clay and allow to dry. Wash and reapply every 2 hours or so until pain and redness goes away.

SPRAINS

Treat sprains both internally and topically as follows:
Days 1-2
Drink 2 ounces liquid Calcium Bentonite Clay twice daily. Apply a ½" thick poultice, large enough to more than cover the area of damage. Leave it on for 30-45 minutes. Reapply 3-4 times daily. At bedtime, coat the affected area with a thin layer of hydrated Calcium Bentonite Clay, allow to dry and

leave on overnight. Take a clay bath daily, immersing the affected area.

Days 3 – until healed

Drink 1 ounce liquid Calcium Bentonite Clay twice daily. Apply a poultice twice a day as indicated above. At bedtime, coat with hydrated Calcium Bentonite Clay and allow to dry, leaving it on overnight.

STRETCH MARKS – see Scars

SUNBURNS – see Burns

SYPHILIS – see Sexually Transmitted Diseases

TATTOO REMOVAL

Tattoo removal using Calcium Bentonite Clay takes 2-6 months, but is a simple, inexpensive, non-invasive method of removing unwanted tattoos.

All ink is of a positive charged ion. Calcium Bentonite Clay is of course a negative charged ionic molecule. Calcium Bentonite Clay literally absorbs and adsorbs the ink out of your skin and it is slowly and progressively washed away.

For the duration of the removal process simply keep a thin layer of hydrated Calcium Bentonite Clay over the tattoo. Leave on at least 1 hour per application and repeat 3-4 times a day. In the evening leave the final application on overnight.

TOENAIL FUNGUS – see Fungus

TONSILLITIS – see Sore Throat

TOOTHACHE

Treat a toothache both internally and topically. Drink 2 ounces of liquid Calcium Bentonite Clay twice daily for the duration of the toothache.

Apply a thick coating of hydrated Calcium Bentonite Clay, or a small poultice, to the outside of your cheek, jaw, or chin, directly over the toothache. Leave on for 45-60 minutes. Repeat 3-5 times daily or until pain/infection is gone. Apply dry powder clay over the tooth. Leave in over night.

TUMORS

To begin treatment for tumors, please first read the section on Cancer and then the section on Detoxification – Full Body. Both contain all of the treatment elements for tumors. Please follow the protocol for detoxification then apply poultices to the specific tumorous areas of your body as described in the Cancer section.

I also want to refer you to the most dramatic series of photos imaginable, along with a 21-day narrative text, showing a doctor removing a tumor from his own body with Calcium Bentonite Clay. Please go to http://silverdata.20m.com/skin-cancer.html and take the time to read every word and study every photo in this series. It truly is a profound documentation of the healing powers of clay and the removal of tumors. I am hopeful this link will remain live for some years to come.

ULCERS

In 1980, Dr. Barry Marshall proved that H pylon bacteria cause many ulcers. Calcium Bentonite Clay not only kills this bacterium, but also contains magnesium and calcium. These are the active ingredients in most over-the-counter medications used to treat heartburn by neutralizing stomach acid and coating sensitive ulcers in the stomach and upper regions of the small intestine. In addition to changes in diet and lifestyle, we suggest drinking 2 to 3 ounces of liquefied Calcium Bentonite Clay three times daily for 21 days. The clay should be taken first thing in the morning, at mid-day and as the last thing consumed at night. After three weeks, continue with a daily maintenance program of consuming one ounce of the liquefied clay at night before bedtime.

There is no faster or more effective cure for ulcers than Calcium Bentonite Clay. The clay helps to alkalize an acid stomach bringing almost instant relief. It also rebuilds the gastrointestinal wall, which has been eaten through by the acid.

UTERINE TUMORS – see Tumors

VARICOSE VEINS

Varicose veins are caused by a toxic blood system. The small, fine capillaries, near the surface of the skin become clogged, stopping blood flow to its spider web looking field of even finer capillaries. These blood toxins normally settle in our lower extremities, our legs, and in later years as toxins build and circulation lessens, varicose and spider veins begin appearing.

Complete a full body detoxification as a first step.

Secondly, drink 1-2 ounces of liquid Calcium Bentonite Clay as a life practice.

Third, soak your legs daily for 2-4 weeks in a clay bath.

Last, apply hydrated Calcium Bentonite Clay topically to the affected areas as you would a thin facial mask. You may "wear" this clay mask as long as you like before washing it off.

VOMITING – See Nausea

WARTS

Warts are usually quickly and easily removed using Calcium Bentonite Clay.

Drink 2 ounces liquid Calcium Bentonite Clay twice daily. Dab on a relatively heavy amount of hydrated Calcium Bentonite Clay directly onto the wart. Leave it on and allow it to dry. Repeat this process 5-6 times daily. At the end of the day, apply the last coating, cover with a cloth bandage and leave on all night.

After 7-14 days you will notice small pieces of the wart beginning to simply flake off as you wash off the clay. Continue the process until the wart is completely gone and smooth skin appears in its place – it could take as long as 30-45 days for larger warts.

Once healed, continue drinking 1 ounce liquid Calcium Bentonite Clay as a daily practice.

WASP STINGS – see Insect Stings

WEIGHT LOSS

You may have come into contact with a hundred diet products and programs, but I'll bet you've never before heard of clay being used as a slimming agent. All over the world, people ingest clay to help acquire and maintain a shapely figure. Sound strange? Earlier I mentioned that clay is typically ingested in famine times to help combat starvation; it temporarily satisfies the hunger and creates a feeling of fullness. For this same reason, clay will keep the weight off. It expands in the stomach, making less room for the food, and thereby relieves the pangs of hunger.

Another advantage to taking clay for weight loss is that it helps to increase the number of bowel movements as well as their quality. Often the weight of waste matter alone is enough to add a few extra pounds to the body. For instance, many of the various diet products on the market contain laxatives to help relieve a constipated condition. Furthermore, clay will assist the assimilation of food. This may, in turn, cut down on the intense need to eat, which may be a sign of malnourishment. Even in an overweight person, if the cells are not having their nutritional needs met, the body can starve to death.

Obesity has become a major health concern for a majority of us. Recent studies indicate that two-thirds of American adults are either overweight or obese. Dr. David Ludwig, director of the Obesity Program at Children's Hospital in Boston states that body weight is affected by many genetic, psychological and environmental factors that influence diet and activity levels. He also says fast food; sugar-sweetened drinks and low-quality junk food have been major contributors to obesity, as have cutbacks in funding for regular, mandatory physical education in schools and limited health coverage for obesity prevention and treatment.

We understand there's a problem, and we understand the health risks. What most people don't understand however, is how to win the weight loss war. Billions are spent each year on fad diets and "miracle" pills that often do more harm than good. We need to understand WHY obesity is on the rise.

What is Causing This Alarming Rise in Obesity?

One of the major contributing factors to obesity is toxins in our bodies. Substances that are toxic to our bodies come at

us from all directions: the air we breathe, the food we eat, the water we drink, the cleaning products we use, and the metabolic waste produced inside us. Toxin build-up in the body contributes to premature aging and chronic and degenerative diseases. Studies have discovered various chemicals from our foods and environment that indicate man contributes 700,000 tons of pollutants into the air every day, ranging from everyday household cleaners to cosmetics and hair dyes. Chemicals and toxins accumulate in fat tissue. The more chemicals and toxins, the more fat the body manufactures.

Another study indicates weight gain and depression are just two common manifestations of a congested, overworked liver. The following are the most common symptoms and conditions: being on edge (easily stressed), elevated cholesterol, skin conditions, skin irritation, depression, sleep difficulties, indigestion, kidney damage, heart damage, brain damage, hypothyroidism, chronic fatigue, weight gain, poor memory, PMS, mental fog, blood sugar disorders, allergies, obesity. If you have tried many ways to improve your health and energy level and nothing seemed to adequately help, it is very possible that your overworked liver underlies your difficulties. Restoring liver function is one of the most important and vital actions you could ever do for your health. When the liver gets congested and toxic, it will remain that way and get worse until it gets detoxified and rejuvenated.

How Can CLAY Help Me Lose Weight?

To lose weight, it's imperative to get rid of the toxins in your body. Nothing is better for this than clay. According to Ran Knishinsky, author of *The Clay Cure*, the best, most natural way to internally cleanse and detoxify is with clay. The following is an excerpt from his book:

"If the system fails to get rid of poisons through the bowels, a constipated condition arises in which the toxins never leave the body. They sit inside and putrefy. What's worse, the body doesn't know the difference between live food and dead food in the colon. It will still try to get nourishment out of waste you would never want to set your eyes upon. Naturally, this puts a strain on every functioning cell in the body.

The clay's immediate action upon the body is directly on the digestive channel. This involves the clay actually binding with the toxic substances and removing them from the body with the stool. It performs this job with every kind of toxin, including those from the environment, such as heavy metals, and those that occur naturally as by-products of the body's own health processes, such as metabolic toxins. It's hard to believe that the body produces its own toxins, but that may happen as a result of stress, inefficient metabolism, or the proliferation of free radicals.

The body has no problem ridding itself of the clay. Don't worry about a tiny brick house being built in the middle of your colon. The clay assists the body's eliminatory process by acting as a bulking agent, similar to psyllium fiber, sweeping out the old matter that doesn't need to be there. It is not digested in the same manner as food as it passes through the alimentary canal. Instead, it stimulates intestinal peristalsis, the muscular contractions that move food and stool through the bowels. The clay and the adsorbed toxins are both eliminated together; this keeps the toxins from being reabsorbed into the bloodstream.

Clay works on the entire organism. No one part of the body is left untouched by its healing energies. I don't know of another supplement that is quite as capable as clay of producing such a wide range of positive reactions."

He goes on to discuss dieting with clay:

"When dieting with clay, the important thing to watch out for is that you don't skip meals or skip out on good nutrition. While the clay helps to satisfy hunger, it doesn't work the same as a "fat burner." It's not going to blast you with caffeine high and enable you to drop pounds quickly."

Drink 2 ounces liquid Calcium Bentonite Clay 3 times a day daily and drink plenty of water. Take 1-2 clay baths weekly. Do 1 full body clay wrap weekly. Continue this treatment regimen until you have reached the desired weight.

WORMS – see Parasites

WOUNDS – TRAUMATIC INJURIES

Traumatic wounds—open bleeding wounds—such as you might see in an auto accident or on the battlefield can be treated with Calcium Bentonite Clay.

Dry powder Calcium Bentonite Clay is anti-microbial and anti-bacterial. It is also highly absorbent and is an excellent clotting agent. If there is an open bleeding wound, simply hand cast, or pack into the wound, dry powder Calcium Bentonite Clay. Use your hand as a pressure bandage and hold closed until the bleeding has stopped or clotted.

Many injuries of an emergency nature will require broken bones to be set, and often both internal and external sutures to be used to close large wounds.

Calcium Bentonite Clay is excellent as a first aid tool and should be available on every ambulance and emergency vehicle in the U.S. Every battlefield soldier should carry it. It should be in every emergency first aid kit on the planet.

Even after a wound is cleaned, sutured and bandaged, Calcium Bentonite Clay used in liquid form internally and poured topically over the sutures and wound itself will quicken the healing process.

YEAST INFECTION

Although a yeast infection has a different causation than Candida, please see that section for treatment. Treatment is the same for both.

What Your Friends and Neighbors Have To Say About Living Clay
Testimonials from real people...

Reading about clay, learning about clay and understanding the science behind clay's efficacy is one thing. Hearing about personal results from your friends or family members is quite another...Then again, using clay and experiencing the miracle of its healing powers yourself constitutes yet quite another level of "understanding."

I am including here a few of my favorite testimonials from that second tier of understanding. These are unsolicited testimonials from real people. My hope is that you will find one that will move you to that third tier of understanding – personal use and your own success story.

They are presented in no particular order and are published as submitted to a leading Calcium Bentonite Clay company, with no editing...

Gulf War Illness—

"I am a gulf war veteran. I was activated January 1991 and had to leave three small children (my oldest was only five). Although I was not deployed to the war zone, I was inoculated with a whole array of vaccines along with everyone else. I spent most of my deployment in England, from where we launched our cargo planes loaded with supplies for the troops in Iraq.

Toward the end of my mobilization, I came down with a serious kidney infection, and when I was demobilized I continued to feel sickly. I was chronically tired, but could never get a restful night's sleep. I had a dull headache all the time, my gums were sore and bleeding, and my joints ached. After my demobilization, I felt as if I had aged fifty years!

I began to pay close attention to my diet, eating as much fresh vegetables and fruits.....getting organic as much as possible. I began supplementing my diet with CoQ10, alpha lipoic acid, milk thistle extract, vitamin c, a good probiotic, and just as much "good stuff" as I could get into my body. These things seemed to help somewhat, but I just couldn't seem to get total and consistent relief from the symptoms I was experiencing.

About two years ago, I accidentally came across the WARL radio station in Providence, which was airing The Power Hour at that time. Working as a structural inspector on a jobsite, I had gotten into my company vehicle to warm up, since it was well below zero outside. I was tired of mainstream propaganda on the radio and started scanning the radio waves, and there was Joyce talking about "real health." After that day, I didn't want to miss one edition of the Power Hour. And when I learned what Joyce and Dave have been doing for vets for so long, it practically brought tears to my eyes, I was so grateful for them!

Anyway, I began using oregano products, coconut oil, essential oils, flax lignan and some other items, which again improved my condition.

Then, one day Joyce had this guest on who was talking about eating dirt every day! I thought "what!?" As I listened to this man describe the many curing abilities of this miraculous "dirt," I made a decision that I was going to get some, as I still was battling bleeding gums, canker sores, and pains in the back of my neck and knee joints.

I started taking one teaspoon of clay with purified water first thing in the morning and before bed. I continued this regimen for about the next nine months, until one day this summer, I went to the beach with my husband and several of our friends for a diving adventure. After diving, we girls went into the ladies room to change and wash the salt and sand off. And as we were washing and chatting in front of the mirrors, one of the ladies looked at me, her eyes with the look of amazement, and she said to me "you have the best skin I've ever seen!" I didn't know what to say except, "Thanks, what a kind thing to say." Then I looked in the mirror and noticed that a liver spot I'd had on my left cheek since my last pregnancy, which was in 1989, about the size of a quarter, which had started to rise at one point, was completely gone! My complexion really was even-toned and radiant! I hadn't even noticed until that lovely comment was made!

What I really noticed, however, since eating clay everyday and using only clay and sea salt as a dentifrice, is a complete clearing of my gum problems, the lack of joint and neck pain, no headaches, and I sleep like a baby! The chronic fatigue I'd lived with for so long had disappeared completely!

Thank you for providing and researching this God-sent substance for those of us who can now use this to heal ourselves and to purify ourselves of the many toxins we ingest knowingly and unknowingly. I do believe this "miracle dirt" could be the key to curing Gulf War Illness and to restoring our many sick veterans (about 260,000) back to health. God bless you all." - Donna D., Master Sergeant, US Air Force, Retired

Cuts, Spider Bites & Rashes —

"Externally, every condition I have applied Calcium Bentonite Clay to has improved dramatically or been cured. Lacerations, bedsores, spider bites, poison ivy and mysterious rashes seem to vanish. In fact, I "discovered" clay when I sliced my fingers open with a razor knife while cutting sheetrock. I sprinkled dry clay onto the cuts and they stopped bleeding within a minute. Then I bandaged them up and went back to work. And then to my great astonishment, within 15 minutes the pain was gone and the cuts completely healed within 3 days. I also used it on a cat bite that wasn't healing (very dangerous) and it cleared up overnight." - Julie C.

Spider Bite – Brown Recluse —

"I had been cutting and stacking wood when I felt a sting on my lower lip. I soon realized from the pain and swelling it must have been a spider bite. Four days and three doctors later, a nurse found the bite mark and determined I had been bitten by a Fiddleback spider (Brown Recluse). By then my lip was about 4 times its normal size and I was sick from the spider's poison. Fiddleback bites can be deadly, often leaving large, open wounds that take many weeks to heal and leave permanent scars. My next-door neighbor gave me some Calcium Bentonite Clay made into a poultice and showed me how to use it. I packed it on my lower face and covered it with lettuce leafs to keep it moist. The following day the pain was receding and my color was returning to normal. My neighbor had gagged at all the infection and dead tissue that came off with the clay pack after just a couple of hours. I continued applying 3 new packs a day and by the next day the swelling was down to half. In 3 days it was completely healed." - Mike B.

Chicken Pox –

"My 22 year old daughter came down with a serious case of chicken pox. She was very ill and covered from head to toe with pox, which nearly drove her crazy because of the itching and irritation. She mixed Calcium Bentonite Clay with water to a very thin film consistency and applied it to her entire body. In a matter of hours the healing set in and she had complete rest and relief. Her recovery was fast and her skin remained lovely – the pox left no scars, which was a miracle." - Kit N.

Psoriasis –

"My doctors said there was no cure for my lifetime battle with psoriasis and gave me a long list of expensive things to buy at the pharmacy suggesting some relief might occur. None of these had worked in the past so I chose to try a natural remedy I had recently heard about. I ordered a pound of Calcium Bentonite Clay, mixed it with water to make a thick paste and applied it to the spots. After it dried completely I gently washed it off with warm water and dried it completely. At night I applied the paste and wrapped my legs in plastic and let it dry more gradually. I began this treatment in August, and by the end of October, only 2 ½ months later, there were no traces of psoriasis left on my body." - Nell C.

Cataracts –

"I was suffering from cataracts and eventual loss of sight and was advised by a psychic to use water filtered through Calcium Bentonite Clay as eye drops, combining this treatment with Calcium Bentonite Clay paste to the eyelids. The treatment was effective and the cataracts completely dissolved." - Karen S

Pyorrhea —

"My pyorrhea finally got so bad my dentist told me all my teeth would need to be extracted. It seemed my teeth were fine but my gums would have to go. I began brushing my teeth and gums with hydrated Calcium Bentonite Clay and packing my gums in the evening at bed time with dry powder. Today, one year later, my teeth are pearly white and my gums are a healthy pink and disease free. All thanks to Calcium Bentonite Clay." - Jim B.

Genital Herpes –

"I had been suffering for 10 years with genital Herpes Simplex – a virus – with monthly outbreaks of blisters on my penis. I have used a very expensive cream prescribed by my doctor, but to no avail, and the outbreak was spreading. I heard about Calcium Bentonite Clay from a web search. I began applying a thin film solution to the affected and surrounding area. Within 3 days all the redness and swelling had disappeared. Within a week all blisters, peeling and necrosis had disappeared. All that remained was fresh pink flesh. No outbreaks occurred for an entire year. When my last outbreak occurred, I nipped it in the bud in 2 days and also began drinking the Calcium Bentonite Clay in a liquid form. Today, 2 years since my last outbreak, after my last blood test for the virus, there is no trace of Herpes virus in my body. I have been cured of Herpes Simplex Virus!" - Carl T.

Blackheads –

"I just got your clay yesterday, and used it as a mask on my face. IMMEDIATELY after rinsing it off, I noticed a HUGE reduction in my blackheads, which I have had problems with for years! WOW!!! I could not believe it. I thought I'd have to use it for a few weeks to see results, but no – literally after the first use there was a huge improvement.

The mask felt great while it was on too. I swear I could feel it working. I was very pleased that you included a free sample of the hydrated clay, because I did not know you had to hydrate the powder for 24 hours, so it was nice to be able to try it out right away (the sample) and then mix some up for use a few days later.

I am incredibly impressed with this product already, and I have already raved about it to a co-worker who has Rosacea. I am bringing her a sample tomorrow. I also thank you for the free samples of the soufflé. I can guarantee you I will be a repeat customer. These products actually do what they say they will do. I am very, very impressed. THANK YOU!" - Kristian

Acne –

"Living Clay...Let me tell you what it has done for me....For the past 24 years, I've had acne along with scarring...it is so embarrassing and humiliating to be in your 40's and still break out. And when I say I've tried everything, for the control of the acne as well as for scar removal, I have tried most of the truly legitimate products that have come on the market and NOTHING has given me the results that your clay has!

I have used everything from Retin-A to professional Dermabrasion and everything in between, and just cannot bring myself to doing a chemical peel or laser surgery.

I take the clay by liquid or capsule once daily and I use the Facial Cleanse to wash my face, then I apply a thin layer of it and use the Wrinkle Release Cream on top of that and once a week I use the hydrated clay as a mask.

I absolutely LOVE this stuff and hope to never be without it! My skin looks better than it has in years and though I still break out occasionally, it is not near with the severity as before and the scarring is beginning to minimize gently and I guess the best part is my skin is not blotchy or ruddy, I don't even wear make-up anymore because I have a natural glow!

I also have to say that I think it is the combination of taking the clay internally as well as using it externally the way I do that has brought such wonderful results.

Thank you everyone at ——————! To know that I am using a product that is so good for me and beneficial is an awesome feeling!

One last thing...the liquid clay is second to none for helping people with any kind of digestive problems, but especially Acid Reflux. I am a Nurse and have given it to several people with this problem and they all beg me for more.

Thanks again....I just wanted you to know that you have helped yet another person in a most magnificent way! - Lori H.

Weight Loss –

"I am doing a Clay facial once in a while. And once in a while I do a Clay bath soak. I am very loyal about drinking it twice a day and taking plenty of water as my only beverage other than Darjeeling and various green teas. When I began drinking a pure natural Calcium Bentonite Clay at the end of January 2005, I drank plenty of water along with the clay. I don't sleep all night so I had a carafe of water handy and each and every time I woke up I drank water. I am not that loyal to doing it lately since I sleep more soundly and wake up fewer times. Consequently, I have not been dropping as fast the additional weight. So there is a clue here. Drink plenty of water.

By Easter at the end of March I realized I was not eating the foil-covered eggs I had purchased for my husband. :-) The clay had just honed down my binges and moderated my desire to eat and over eat. I am satisfied with better food and much smaller portions. The candy section and the bakery section holds NO temptation for me now. I do not feel like I have to be putting drink or food into my system all the time as I did before drinking the clay. Water being the only exception. I always have a bottle of water at the ready. My shape change came about without effort. I did not exercise; I do feel now like I could. I have fibromyalgia and related health problems, so exercising was not for me. At first my shape change was subtle. I noticed my clothes getting comfortable, that was a surprise since my washer and dryer (Maytag) has always shrunk my clothes. Then they just didn't stay on my hips. My arms and shoulders no longer fit the shirts and blouses and the shoulder pads I once tossed out would be needed to continue to wear them. My guess is that I am not being controlled by the parasites who had been supported by the chemicals and other trash in what I had been consuming. The clay did its job and cleaned them out. The only other changes I made was getting a mercury filling taken out and dropping all medications. Both had long been on my mind to do and clay had just given me the vehicle to carry away the residue/toxins that my "habits" or poor judgment had left behind. The truth at last, a pure natural Calcium Bentonite Clay is effective and harmless at the same time. Will I ever stop drinking clay twice a day? After going from 3x and 2x to size 14 (for now) I will always drink clay." - Linda R.

Multiple Uses-

I started using the Living Clay about 6 months after Linda (see Linda R. above). Of course seeing what it was doing for Linda was proof enough for me (I guess one would say I am a bit skeptical and have to see results). I lost my father to cancer and then my mother was diagnosed with colon cancer and beat it after having surgery. Her doctor said her children should be checked out no matter what our ages so 3 years ago I went in for the dreaded colonoscopy and I had a polyup they said could turn to cancer so they said to come back in three years (this year). I recently had my second colonoscopy and I was clean...!!! I completely attribute this to the living clay but some might think otherwise...!

In my job, I travel normally 3 weeks out of 4 every month. One day I was extremely late for the airport (not wanting to get stuck in the security checks), and as I past a pizzeria heading for my gate, I darted in for a hot slice of pizza (very unusual as I strive to eat organic and healthy). Not thinking (because my stomach was rumbling) I pulled it out of the box and bit into this VERY HOT slice of cheese pizza. Needless to say, the hot cheese welded itself to the roof of my mouth and burned it terribly. For the next 3 hours on the plane, I couldn't even drink water without it hurting and the pain seemed to be intensifying. When I arrived at my location and checked into my room, I decided to get my bottle of clay out and drink some. The results were unbelievable...the pain, soreness, throbbing was instantly gone...and never returned...!!! There is no other explanation for what happened except the living clay stopped the blistering and pain related to a burn and healed my mouth.

About 18 months ago, a co-worker had to have his prostrate removed. At his one year check up things looked clean but he still had to have blood work accomplished every 3 months. In January of this year, he approached me and said even though he didn't have a prostrate anymore, his PSA was climbing. I asked how could this be and he said the doctors told him the cancer seems to collect in the area where the prostrate used to be which is seen by the elevated PSA count. I immediately gave him my supply of hydrated clay and told him to start drinking 4 oz in the morning and at night (boy did I miss my clay, but it was worth it). Two weeks later he went back for more blood work and his PSA was down and in the green.

Recently, I had another chance to see what the Living Clay has accomplished in another person's life. I have an individual in the office who was having problems sleeping and went to the medical community for help. After giving her a complete physical and finding nothing "out of sorts," they decided MRI (from the top of her head to mid-chest) to see if it would show anything. Well it did...but it was not associated with what they were looking for...! They found an enlarged lymph node next to her heart by the aorta. She was told they wanted to check it out in another two weeks...well needless to say she was terrified...!!! She came and talked to me and I immediately told her to order some of the Living Clay powder which she did! Linda mailed her some over night to hold her over until her order arrived. I instructed her how to use it...she bathed in it and drank it for about 4 or 5 days before she was scheduled for her CT (from the bottom of the head to lower abdomen). The doctor wanted the same radiologist who read the MRI to read the CT and had to wait a few days before calling her with the results. The Doctor started out saying they now thought it was just an inflamed lymph node because it was smaller from when they first had seen it in the MRI. Then the doctor asked if she had been taking Pepto Bismal...curious at to what initiated the question...my friend said no...why do you ask? The doctor said the CT showed the entire intestinal track was lined with something like Pepto Bismal...!!! My friend then said she had been drinking calcium bentonite clay! The doctor said she had heard about it, what it was and to keep taking it because it is good for you...!!! Now you can come to your own conclusion but personally, knowing what I know...seeing what I have seen...I personally feel the clay immediately started to reverse the problem with the lymph node...and I think the doctor did as well but since she is a mainstream doctor, and a military one too...I feel she couldn't give the real reason as to what had occurred with my friends health...!!!!

Dan R.

Acne Prevention –

"I've been using the clay on my face for about a year. My skin is clearer and at the first site of a breakout, the clay goes on. I often sleep with a light layer for maintenance, which really aids in prevention of acne. I've thrown out all other products and have saved a ton of money!!" - Heather D.

Psoriasis and Energy Level –

"I have been using clay for about a month now, in that month I have noticed an increase in my energy, I feel better. I also have noticed that all my psoriasis has disappeared completely, I tried cortisone creams for years. My friends and husband have noticed a brighter appearance in my face. I am so thankful for your clay and plan to keep using it the rest of my life. I have told many of my friends about your product." - Marsha R.

Abscessed Tooth –

"What a miracle! I had an abscessed tooth and was beginning to get the toxins spread into my throat and my ears. I called my sister-in-law to see what she thought I should do. I can't take antibiotics, as they always seem to cause me problems and was not prepared to deal with that again. She had just purchased the clay in powder form and ran some over to me to try. Within two hours after applying a paste to my abscess it had drawn the infection out. I continued to apply the paste that night and the next day to fully heal the tooth and I was infection free. Since the clay worked so well on my tooth I decided to use it for a mask on my face and wow what a difference it made in my skin. Needless to say I am in the process of purchasing my own clay." - Laura G.

Acne –

"When my son, Ryan, hit puberty his face erupted with acne. The poor kid had it so bad that you could hardly see his face underneath all the zits. I took him to a dermatologist who wanted to prescribe an oral medication. Because I know the havoc taking medication can have on the body I was against that. Next the doctor prescribed a topical ointment of Rentin A, this caused his skin to turn bight red and it became extremely painful in the sunshine. Imagine an active teenage boy who loves to ski, play in the pool with his brothers and soccer with his friends, hiding inside all day because even to walk outside was too painful. To occupy his time inside he spent a lot of time in front of the TV or the computer, this started to cause a little chubbiness around his middle. Now not only was his face literally peeling off and bright red – it looks worse than just the acne, he was becoming an introverted couch potato. The clay was introduced to us last year and after just a few weeks of using just the clay daily as a mask, Ryan's acne has for the most part cleared up, he is back outside enjoying his life and we are not paying an arm and a leg for prescriptions." - Angie F.

Cleanse –

"I love your products so much! I first heard about your clay on *The Power Hour*. The 2 hours he spent on the show were absolutely fascinating and the clay is superb. I eat it twice daily &

apply it externally as well. I feel more energized, my eye whites are clearer and my digestive system is running so much better. I am telling everybody about your website & your great products. My sons love what it has done for their acne. I have also tried it (very successfully) on my younger sons dandruff problem. I added some hydrated clay to his shampoo and the dandruff is gone. I think there are almost unlimited possibilities for using your clay. I am so grateful." - Louise J.

Hair Growth –

"Thanks again for your service and the privilege to share my story. In August of 1999, three weeks short of my nineteenth birthday, I was diagnosed with Leukemia. During my first round of chemotherapy, my thick dark brown hair fell out as a side effect often found with chemotherapy patients. Over the course of my treatments, my hair would often grow back between rounds of chemotherapy in unusual ways, such as blonde and light brown. At the end of my cancer treatment, I underwent a bone marrow transplant that left me bald once again. Before I continue, I would like to say that I am blessed and proud to say that I am cancer free, and that beating cancer will not be the biggest accomplishment in my life. Still, as a young man in his early twenties, my self-image still plays a role in my confidence and over the last four years, since the transplant, my hair has yet to return to its original dark thickness. A year after the transplant, my hair began to grow back in light thin peach fuzz on the sides but nothing on the top.

My doctors stated that perhaps like my father I was going bald and it just happened to occur at the same time as my treatment. As the weeks and months continued, my hair began to thicken in certain areas at times, but at an extremely slow rate. I began to shave my head because in my opinion, if I didn't it appeared more like I was losing my hair rather then the fact it was growing back. Extremely frustrated at the rate of hair growth I was experiencing, early this past summer I questioned if my hair would ever return. A trip to the oncologist lead to a blood test which revealed that all my hormonal levels associated with balding men were normal. Baffled for an explanation, I was referred to a famous dermatologist in Manhattan who specialized in hair loss. His "diagnosis" was that I was going bald and he recommended some oral and topical medications to keep the little hair I had. I didn't agree with his diagnosis and it didn't make sense to believe that I was balding when every few months I was getting a few new hairs here and there.

Last August I was exposed to this amazing clay from a friend who recommended that I give it a try for my scalp. I began using the clay in September and in the last three months the results are INCREDIBLE! Less than one month into using the clay topically once a day people began to notice the increase of hair. The rate of dark thick hair growth is compounding each week. I now have a date at which I expect a full head of hair that is less then a year thanks to this amazing clay where six months ago I began to doubt if that would ever be possible again. With my most recent order, I now plan to ingest the clay as well for the benefit of my health *and* my hair. Thank you for providing such an outstanding product from such an outstanding and caring customer service team! - Michael I.

Ant Bites –

"On my February 2004 missionary trip to New Hope Mission in Uganda, Africa, I took some Calcium Bentonite Clay for my sister to try. While there a vicious ant similar to our infamous Texas Fire ants stung me. I remembered reading about the benefits of using it on insect bites so I decided to give it a try. Wow was I glad I did! Within several seconds the burning and itch began to subside and within a minute was completely gone. The next day there was no small pimple as usual with ant stings and after reapplying the clay the sting mark was gone the next day. It also worked great to soothe the mosquito bites.

Thanks for sharing the many uses of this great product on your website. PS My mom and sister like using the clay because it really pulls out the toxins and helps their face feel and look better." - Michael M.

Poison Oak –
"Yesterday, I was introduced to Calcium Bentonite Clay to help a severe case of poison oak. I applied a small amount of the clay directly on the poison oak and in 24 hours it was dried up and was almost gone. It did not take long to see the healing results. I feel so much better!" - Michael F.

Acne –
"My daughter has fought with acne for two years. We'd tried every over-the-counter remedy on the market, and nothing worked. A friend told us about Calcium Bentonite Clay, and we decided to give it a try. My daughter began applying the clay once a day, letting it dry, and then washing it off. At first, she experienced some redness, but we were told to expect that, so she kept using it. Within 1 week, her face was clear of pimples, and within two weeks, there weren't even any red marks left! I've never seen her so happy! Thank you!" Martha B.,

Itchy skin and Loose Bowels -
My daughter is nine years old. We thought she had allergies or ADHD or something because she was always moving. I finally asked her why she moved all the time and she said she was itchy. I even used the Lubriderm lotion thinking it was dry skin and she reacted to that as well. The clay soap for bath time and the lotion I had originally bought for myself did the trick. My husband uses the clay and his loose bowels have corrected and he reports more volume as well. We are going to start my daughter on the clay capsules. We're fans! Andrea B.

Heartburn and Indigestion –

"I'm very skeptical about new products, but I'm quickly becoming a believer in Calcium Bentonite Clay. I've suffered with heartburn and indigestion for years and years, and have been using Prevacid as needed – usually 2-3 times a week. Last week, I ran out of my Prevacid, and had a nasty case of heartburn late at night. My wife brought me some of her liquid clay. I tried it, and almost instantly the heartburn was gone. I'm a believer in results, and this stuff gets results." - Phillip E.

Underarm Nodules –

I just personally witnessed another miracle with Calcium Bentonite Clay. I had a client that I had been working on for 2 ½ years (ear coning and colonics). Under her arms were these red bumps that itched. The skin would peel from this area. She said she'd had this for as long as she could remember. She had never gone to a doctor. Just before moving from Los Angeles, I worked on her several times utilizing ear coning and colonics.

I moved to Charlotte, NC with my arms full of red itchy bumps. At night they seemed to get overwhelmingly itchy. One time I scratched so hard I drew blood.

I use tea tree oil as a deodorant and I could no longer use it because it now stung. I first covered my underarms topically with the hydrated clay and it felt so cool and soothing. It would stop the itching temporarily. After doing this a couple of times I noticed the areas under my arms had begun clearing up. That night I took 4 clay capsules then two more soon after I went to bed. I was also bathing in the clay powder.

That night I went through something emotional. I awoke the next morning and noticed my underarms had cleared up even more over night. The next day, I took 6 more capsules. The horrific rash of bumps was almost completely gone! Incredible. Still some slight itching. The 3rd day I took 4 capsules and a clay bath. I have also been using your soap and brushing my teeth with the clay.

My underarms are free of bumps and itching and the horrible uncomfortable madness is gone. That is one thing I could identify that energetically got passed from my client to me! I wonder how many other things I am holding that my clients have released that I'm not aware of.

I think Calcium Bentonite Clay is excellent protection for practitioners that work in others energy. Amazing. I feel soooo much better.

Clay…God's gift to mankind. Cynthia L.

Hand Rash-

It was my sister's birthday so I bought her some Bentonite clay. When I brought her present to her I had also given her a small sample of the clay which had already been prepared. Just a day prior to my visit, my sister broke out with tiny pus-like pimples all over both of her hands. Not only did her hand look "diseased" but she complained terribly about the itch. I was so happy I had provided her with a prepared sample along with her present. I urged her to immediately apply the clay to her hands and within a half hour the itching had subsided. I told her to use it as often as possible and she told me within a couple of days the rash had disappeared.

We don't know exactly what caused this skin outbreak but apparently it was an allergic reaction to something. The calcium Bentonite clay eradicated the problem. Imagine—no waiting in the doctor's office, no harmful drugs with side affects. This product is wonderful!!

Thank you
Gail P.

THE FDA AND
CALCIUM BENTONITE CLAY

During a recent FDA compliance review of product labeling of a well-known Calcium Bentonite Clay company, an issue arose regarding their weight statement on their 1 pound jars of dry powder Calcium Bentonite Clay. For years the company had shown the weight as 'Net Wt. 16 oz.' It seems the FDA guidelines consider this to be confusing to the consumer and sent the following statute to the company to help them better understand how the FDA required weights to be shown on containers. Further, that until the company brought this label and a few others into compliance, all the existing product – wrongly labeled – would be held in detention and could not be sold…

21 CFR 701.13(j)(1-2)

"…the container must bear an accurate statement of the net quantity of contents of the product in the container in terms of weight, measure, numerical count, or a combination of numerical count and weight or measure. The declaration must be distinct, placed in the bottom area of the panel in line generally parallel to the base on which the package rests, and in a type size commensurate with the size of the container as prescribed by regulation 21 CFR 701.13(c). The net quantity of contents statement of a solid, semisolid, or viscous cosmetic must be in terms of the avoidupois pound and ounce, and a statement of liquid measure must be in terms of the U.S. gallon of 231 cubic inches and the quart, pint and fluid ounce subdivisions thereof. The declaration shall appear as a distinct item on the principal display panel, shall be separated (by at least a space equal to the height of the lettering used in the declaration) from other printed label information appearing above or below the declaration and (by at least a space equal to twice the width of the letter "N" of the style of type used in the quantity of contents statement) from other printed label information appearing to the left or right of the declaration. If the net quantity of contents is one pound or more or one pint or more, it must be expressed in ounces, followed in parenthesis () by a declaration of the largest whole units (i.e., pounds and ounces or quarts or pints and ounces). The net quantity of contents may additionally be stated in terms of the metric system of weights or measures…"

Well, as you can imagine, that cleared things right up…About as clear as the "mud" the company was selling!

What the company learned after paying an FDA compliance attorney over $1,000.00 to review this one single statue and to interpret the hieroglyphics, found the label need to read as follows:

"Net Wt. 16 oz. (1 lb.)"

We can only assume the "(1 lb.)" added notation is for the protection of those among us who may believe that 16 oz. is somehow more or less than a pound…Thank God for the FDA and the lengths to which they will go in order to protect us from the obvious pitfalls of such a potential misunderstanding.

Possibly at some point around the time of its inception, the FDA really did serve the good of the people. But as with every good bureaucracy comes the time when the preservation and expansion of the agency becomes its own albatross. And shortly after that comes the money and control of that agency by the very companies it initially set out to protect the citizens from…And that's just where we find ourselves today, with an agency whose initial oversight involved regulatory issues and public health issues over such companies as Bayer who wanted to sell its Aspirin in America.

Around the turn of the century, all things "natural" in the health industry were a good thing. We felt it would serve the public good to monitor and do oversight on the new Pharmaceutical companies, which were creating drugs that were synthesized and made from things known to be toxic to the human body. Simply put, it was the new "poison" pharmaceutical companies that needed the oversight.

Oh, how we've come 180 degrees since those days. Today the FDA is controlled by legislation funded by those poison companies. The FDA board is elected by the FDA Pharmaceutical Company Oversight Committee. In short, the pharmaceutical companies own and operate every aspect of FDA operations. Today the FDA is spending 60% of its resources on investigation and closure of companies marketing purely natural remedies such as herbs and nutrients. It's a complete flip from its initial purpose and one so blatant I often wonder how we all went so deeply asleep at the wheel.

Here's an excerpt from some commentary by Jason Eaton, a well known expert on healing with Calcium Bentonite Clay, describing the fine line we must walk today, and how if crossed, the FDA unleashes its police powers through sister agencies. Keep in mind while reading this excerpt, he is discussing how you may and may not talk about Calcium Bentonite Clay on his Yahoo Groups chat group site. This is how far things have come...

"On our discussion list, we can discuss the science of clays, and certainly share personal experience, and even debate and explore the potential effects. Giving direct medical advice can get an individual in a world of trouble in our country! As for marketing pursuits, you can make no claims without scientific evidence. If you have clear scientific evidence, you can present it. However, even here you have to approach the area with great caution. The FDA does not consider scientific evidence good enough to allow medical claims to be made about natural products. However, the FTC does. The FTC is often the strong arm that the FDA uses to prosecute companies making "unjustified" medical claims. Therefore if you are following guidelines that the FTC recognizes it will be more difficult for the FDA to go after you. Once the FDA does decide to step in, they don't usually care about the law at all, only in shutting you down and forcing compliance. They will bring in the FTC, the IRS, and even attempt, if all else fails, to nail you on postal fraud. (These cases are, of course, when a company stands up for its rights and decides to fight them.) Never ever make any medical claims. A medical claim is defined as using a substance to treat any medical condition (any ailment). Thus stating that Calcium Bentonite Clay sorpts toxins in the body, including specific bacteria, heavy metals, etc., can be lawful...but stating that taking Calcium Bentonite Clay internally cures a stomachache is illegal and you can be sent to prison and have your business seized. The only safe way to discuss natural curative products such as Calcium Bentonite Clay is to never make any curative or medical claims, but provide customers with outside resources that they can research themselves, independent of any actual product marketing."

It's clear that the battle lines have been drawn between the naturalists and the pharmaceutical companies. Lying right in the middle of the battlefield is Calcium Bentonite Clay. It is not only the single most effective, broad spectrum, natural curative, it is also the single most used natural additive to pharmaceuticals...and it is protected by the FDA's GRAS (Generally Recognized As Safe) certification. Both sides claim it as their own. Today there is a very good concern that the availability of Calcium Bentonite Clay will go away. What is in question is whether it will remain available OTC with no regulatory controls or it will become a prescription item only. Let's take a look at the recent FDA ruling regarding Bentonite and its being granted blanket GRAS status as a food and pharmaceutical additive.

CFR Title 21, Vol. 3, Dated April 1, 2005

Part 184 – Direct food substances affirmed as Generally Recognized As Safe

Subpart B – Listing of Specific Substances Affirmed as GRAS

Sec. 184.1155 Bentonite

(a) Bentonite (A1 20, CAS Reg. No. 1302-0978-099) is principally a colloidal hydrated aluminum silicate. Bentonite contains varying quantities of iron, alkalines, and alkaline earths in the commercial products. Depending on the cations present, natural deposits of Bentonite range in color from white to gray, yellow, green or blue. Bentonite's fine particles provide large total surface area and, hence, pronounced adsorptive capability.

(b) FDA is developing food-grade specifications for Bentonite in cooperation with the National Academy of Sciences. In the interim, the ingredient must be of suitable purity for its intended use.

(c) In accordance with 184.1 (b)(1), the ingredient is used in food with no limitation other than current good manufacturing practice. The affirmation of this ingredient as GRAS (Generally Recognized As Safe) as a direct human food ingredient is based upon current good manufacturing practice conditions.

(d) Prior sanctions for this ingredient different from the uses established in this section do not exist or have been waived. [47 FR 43367, Oct. 1, 1981]

Although everyone agrees this GRAS Certification by the FDA is a step in the right direction, it does not solve the problem at hand. What's warranted is a declaration by the FDA that not only is Calcium Bentonite Clay safe as a food "additive," it is safe all by itself in its natural form.

The other FDA recognized certifications are USP (United States Pharmacopoeia) and NF (National Formulary). If Bentonite clay is labeled as meeting USP or NF or USP/NF standards, that means the clay has been cleaned or purified by either a heat or hydration process. These are the only two processes which will lower the microbial counts of Natural

Living Clay enough to be "legally" used and marketed for internal use in medicines or added to creams or lotions for topical use.

While natural unprocessed Calcium Bentonite Clay (Living Clay) is by far the most effective and broad spectrum healer on our planet, the FDA insists it be made to fit its standards of use, required of poisons and other pharmaceuticals; wherein microbial counts above a certain fixed level, about 500 CFU/g, can dramatically affect the viability of a traditional medicine. Therefore, for Calcium Bentonite Clay to be sold in a hydrated form, a liquid form, or as an additive to cosmetics, it must first be "cleansed" of a percentage of its efficacy by removing part of what makes it a Living Clay.

The third standard is FDA/USDA Food Grade certified clay. This "FDA Grade" clay has been nuked with gamma rays almost to a state of no efficacy.

Of the three standards – USP, NF and FDA Grade – only USP retains enough of its natural microbes and healing properties to be used as a hydrated product or additive to cosmeceuticals.

Here is what Jason Eaton has to say on the subject of cleaned or modified clays:

"FDA Grade clay may or may not maintain the healing potency of natural and USP grade clay. These clays tend to be over processed. When we submitted two samples of clay for lab analysis, one FDA grade and one natural, the group doing the analytical work elected not to even study the FDA grade clay after preliminary work using Transmission Electron Microscopy. The highly processed clay was described as useless mud! To qualify this statement, FDA grade clay (and other "purified" clays) will still maintain their ability to absorb substances, and thus may still be sufficient for internal cleansing programs. Needless to say, our recommendation is to use a natural or USP grade Calcium Bentonite Clay for internal use.

One clay processing company which sells various forms of Bentonite for both industrial and pharmaceutical use, markets a standard, unprocessed, 325 mesh, technical grade sodium Bentonite that works better than any other so-called sodium based healing clay that I have tested. No clay company can recommend its clay for use on the body and make healing claims and be in compliance with the FDA guidelines that regulate that segment of the industry. What you need to look for is the USP grade certification or even better—a natural, unaltered Calcium Bentonite Clay.

For internal use, this company sells a USP, pharmaceutical grade Bentonite clay that the FDA has approved for use in the human body. While they do not sell directly to the public, look for a retailer or Internet company that sells both a pure, natural Calcium Bentonite Clay and also their USP grade Bentonite in hydrated and liquid form. The USP grade is also used in creams, lotions, and all kinds of cosmeceuticals."

For the time being, taking into account the nature of the beast we are dealing with, my best advice is to learn to be a smart consumer. You cannot count on the government or the FDA to do your bidding for you.

In support of the preceding paragraph, I want to share with you another interesting sign of the times – the "Public Service Warnings" published by the FDA, whose purpose is to warn consumers about the dangers of natural and herbal products now on the market. The below advisory letter is one of those and was published on November 21, 2003. As you read, please keep in mind this is for the "protection of the consumer."

"Dietary Supplements Containing Herbal Products"

Many Americans view herbal and natural dietary supplements as useful therapeutic agents for treating a wide variety of ailments. Indeed, many effective prescription drugs are derived from plant sources and are proven to be quite effective. Yet, the risks are clear with natural poisons such as hemlock, strychnine and belladonna.

Many people assume that "natural" products are inherently safe and that they may be taken without risk. However, natural products come with a full range of potential risks, as do some synthetic products. Many natural dietary supplements are potentially quite harmful.

Currently, natural dietary and herbal supplement products are unregulated. Consumers who wish to rely on natural dietary or herbal supplements should educate themselves about the risks associated with the products. It is also advisable to develop a healthy skepticism for information on the Internet.

Here are a few guidelines to consider:

"Natural" does not necessarily mean "safe."

Natural dietary and herbal supplements are not miraculous "cure-alls." If a claim sounds too good to be true, it probably is. Beware of sensational names, claims and other misinformation.

If you eat a normal diet, following the Department of Agriculture's Food Guide Pyramid, you should not need additional vitamins, minerals or dietary supplements.

Natural and herbal supplements can interact with prescription drugs and cause harmful effects.

Don't use herbs to self-treat serious or persistent medical conditions.

Don't use herbs or natural dietary supplements if you are pregnant or nursing or give to infants or children under 12 without consulting with your medical doctor.

Homeopathy is a natural health practice whose products utilize little or no active ingredients.

If you have an adverse reaction to any natural or herbal supplement, stop its use immediately and contact a licensed healthcare professional. Report all adverse reactions to the FDA MEDWATCH Adverse Event Monitoring System.

I don't know about you, but I feel safer knowing the FDA is really looking out for me...

In spite of the FDA's scare tactics, there really is a safe and intelligent approach to be taken when shopping for "natural products." I recommend the following:

Learn to read labels, and more importantly, know what those labels mean in relation to your health. Look for a pure, clean, natural, Calcium Bentonite Clay. Look for one with a pH of at least 9.5. If you do internet searches for products, I recommend your initial parameters be "Calcium Bentonite Clay" then read all you care to and determine for yourself what to purchase for health purposes. Consider buying this natural Living Clay in powder form and learn to mix and hydrate it yourself for personal use. It's inexpensive when purchased in small bulk quantities of 4 or 8 pound containers. When buying cosmeceuticals look for a clean, natural Calcium Bentonite Clay or USP grade for use in formulating these wonderful total body care products.

MONATOMICS AND CLAYTRONICS

As science evolves, new words come into our vocabulary. I heard about Monatomics for the first time about 3 years ago when watching a DVD on the subject. The term Claytronics came into my world about 1 short year ago. Both represent the future of Living Clay science.

Monatomic Elements, or "Monatomics," is the technical term for a recently branded form of matter consisting of "orbitally rearranged monatomic elements" – or its acronym of "ORMES." Simply put, and I'm sure you remember I like keeping things simple, these are elements whose atomic orbits have been altered, having thrown off their positive charged proton and now circle the neutron in an elliptical fashion. They now act quite differently than their complete and whole counterparts.

During the past 15 years, researchers have rediscovered this previously hidden form of matter. There are many historical references to monatomic ORMES, which will be discussed shortly, and date to Egyptian and Vedic texts. ORMES, in their most pure and natural form, are found in Calcium Bentonite Clay - Living Clay. This form of matter has been shown to provide tremendous benefits in the field of human health, nutrition, longevity, energy, intuition and spiritual connection.

Monatomic elements are naturally produced by thermal-chemical reactions within the earth's core and spewed forth as fine volcanic ash during volcanic eruptions. Although they can be found in trace amounts virtually anywhere on the earth's surface, they are primarily concentrated in volcanic soils.

In recent years, several proprietary methods of recovering or separating monatomic elements from volcanic soil have been developed. Some claim to have patented their modern alchemy processes but I have been unsuccessful in locating any

141

approved patents on these processes. Most claim their processes to be "trade secrets."

What is common to all of these new researchers is that they offer for sale small vials of a white liquid sold under various trade names at extremely inflated prices. What I believe they have done is to take a specific type of volcanic ash, a Calcium Bentonite Clay, and synthesized out all minerals with the exception of a specific group of metals – gold, platinum, iridium, rhodium, osmium, ruthenium and palladium. Using brand names such as White Powder Gold, Ormus White Gold, and Manna Tonic, prices range from $49 to $199 per fluid ounce. The same volcanic ash, in its natural form, containing these ORMES and other viable minerals can be obtained in a suspended colloidal liquid form for less than $2 per fluid ounce when you purchase Calcium Bentonite Clay.

Monatomic Elements were known in ancient times under different names. Their existence was rediscovered and popularized in the late 1980's by David Hudson an Arizona farmer invested in the mono-dipoly atomic forms of numerous transition metals. When these ORMES first began to be isolated through an acid burn and heating process, the cost of producing these elements was very high. Although various products are currently offered under the name of "monatomic," the majority of these products represent low-grade, over-priced forms of this material.

The most concentrated known sources of monatomic elements are some specific Calcium Bentonite Clay volcanic ash deposits in Death Valley, California. After years of research, a specific volcanic deposit of Living Clay has been identified and a breakthrough in the commercial production of monatomic elements from that deposit has been achieved, in turn making these elements much more affordable.

All monatomic elements consist of inert minerals that are also present in many food substances and herbs, and as a result are already present in the body. Due to their chemical inactivity – the pure negative charged inert atom – they do not assimilate or react within the body like ordinary metal ions or atoms. In addition, in the monatomic state they are completely non-toxic and harmless.

It has been discovered that certain monatomic elements have the potential to assume what is referred to as the "high-spin-state." This refers to a phenomenon discovered in the late 1980's by nuclear physicists at a number of renowned laboratories around the world. They discovered that when certain monatomic metal atoms were put into a high-spin state, the elementary particles inside the nucleus became rearranged and spin around at an increased rate of speed.

As a result of the rearranged orbits, their electromagnetic emissions coming from the high-spin elements are different from the norm. (Scientific American, Oct. 1991, pg. 26, Dr. Philip Yam) It now appears that Nature has its own low-tech, low-energy method of producing these monatomic elements deep within the earth. The miracle of the gift is shared with us through volcanic eruption and the ash left for the use by all, pure, natural Calcium Bentonite Clay.

When ingested in the body in a liquid colloidal form the monatomic elements pervade the body. Because they are chemically inert, the effects cannot be due to any chemical reactions in the body. All benefit is due to the ionic exchange, the energetic effect. Monatomic elements simply reside in the cells, where they generate the subtle essence of life. By enhancing the energy level and balance of the body at a cellular level, more spiritual intelligence can be expressed through both the mind and body.

I recommend daily ingestion of Monatomic elements in their all-natural form of Calcium Bentonite Clay – the Living Essence of Life.

CLAYTRONICS AND CLAYATOMICS

Step into the future. What if there were a form of silica, readily available, that had even greater conductivity than the silicon used in the manufacturing process of all computer CPU's today? And what if that silica was self-cooling, and could transfer data at 1,000+ times the speed of today's norm? And what if that same silica had the inherent organic ability to act more like our biological brain than a binary piece of hardware, such as today's computer brains?

These questions are no longer simply questions. Today these concepts are past the theoretical scientific model. They are proven and they are becoming tomorrow's reality. Living Clay is all the buzz in the futurists' labs. The computer chip giants and worlds foremost robotics experts are moving toward creating a functional living cell "brain-chip."

Intel's robotics expert, Jason Campbell, says, "The more you look at it, the more likely it seems we will be able to manufacture these things on a consumer level."

Scientists in the United States are today developing TINY robots, made from Living Clay that can transform themselves into any shape – from a replica human, to a banana, to a cell phone...

The new science of "Claytronics" which uses nanotechnology to create tiny robots called "Catoms" will enable three-dimensional copies of people to be "faxed" around the world for virtual meetings. A doctor could consult with a patient over the phone, even taking their pulse by holding the wrist of the "Claytronic replica patient," reports New Scientist Journal.

The creator, Dr. Todd Mowry, director of Intel's research labs in Pittsburg, Pennsylvania, said, "You could have a little lump of this stuff you carry around and it could be a million different things. It's the worlds ultimate Swiss Army knife." His partner, Dr. Seth Goldstein, of Carnegie Mellon University in Pittsburg, said, "It's absolutely going to work. Now whether that's 4 or 20 years down the road for consumer use, I don't know."

With Claytronics, millions of tiny individual devices "Claytronic Atoms or Catoms" – would assemble into full-scale objects, connecting and disconnecting as they move. The current, large, proof-of-concept catoms measuring 4 centimeters each, connect and move through electromagnet impulse, much like the "Replicating Robots" devised by Cornell University, only a month prior, which when energized appeared to be a person. Made of millions of tiny micro robots it actually looked like a person. Taking things one-step forward; Goldstein and Mowry see Claytronics as a way of being multiple places at once.

Goldstein and Mowry refer to the larger context of "Transmittable synthetic Reality" as "pario," Latin for "Create and bring forth." They describe their efforts today as being in the infancy stage and are remarkably timid when futurizing about the future of this science. Creating a living, programmable matter is as much of a leap over silicon hardware CPU information as was going from the quill tip pen to digital image printing. There simply is no comparable scientific leap in our history, which compares to the hurdle we are surpassing today.

Scientists at Xerox PARC have been secretly working on Living Clay modalities for several years as well. They call their creations "Smart Matter" or "Digital Clay." One of their primary objectives is to make robotics with multiple mobilities. "Imagine," said a senior research scientist at Xerox, "a search and rescue robot that can roll, slither, or walk depending on any terrain or obstacle encountered."

This technology is still in its infancy, but promises the potential to profoundly affect humanity for many decades to come.

WHERE MONATOMICS AND CLAYTRONICS MEET

The most effective form of Calcium Bentonite Clay consists of 3 primary minerals:

Silica

Calcium

Magnesium

It is no coincidence that in the human body the three most common minerals are as follows:

Silica

Calcium

Magnesium

Living Clay virtually replicates the Living Body in its mineral composition.

When we look at the human brain we find that it is silica that acts as the organic carrier of electrical impulses causing the brain to function, to compute, to cause action, thought, emotion, etc.

When we look at Catom or Claytronics Chip, "CPU's" made from Living Clay, it is the silica that acts as the organic carrier of impulses, causing the CPU to function, to compute, to cause action, thought, emotion, etc.

While traditional binary synthetic silicon based CPU can't experience or create emotion or bilateral reasoning, a Living Clay "Catom" can. This new science is the bridge between hardware and biology. Scientists are literally creating Living Chips!

In addition to silica being the transfer modality of electrical and neurochemical information exchange, monatomic elements also play a role. Analysis shows that the brain tissue of cows may consist of up to 5% of monatomic elements, particularly rhodium and iridium.

The primary function of these monatomic metal elements is greater conductivity and connectivity resulting in increased alpha wave activity. In humans this would amount to a better functioning cerebral colossum, which transfers information between the left and right hemisphere of the cerebellum. This correlates to increased learning ability, improved memory and greater creativity. It may also be argued that the end result would be a more coherent consciousness, an expanded sense of spirituality and heightened intuition.

It is important to note that David Hudson recently went out of business citing his inability to mass produce/extract Monatomics from his source of volcanic ash. He also cited that his own serious health problems and numerous EPA violations regarding his extraction process as reason for ceasing operations. He sent out a letter to all of the people participating and investing in his quest stating he had to abandon all work on his MAE project permanently. He has not commented or appeared in public since that letter was made public.

Calcium Bentonite clay is the "magic stuff" of our collective futures. Calcium Bentonite Clay is believed to be the ultimate source for natural Monatomics. Calcium Bentonite Clay is the body, mind and spirit of Claytronics. Calcium Bentonite Clay is the ultimate curative for the human body. Calcium Bentonite Clay holds the key to all of life itself. As the world reawakens to its curative properties, science comes alive with the discovery, which will propel our society from the computer age to the Claytronics age…

Have you had your clay today?

RECIPES
Yes, you can cook with it, too!

Calcium Bentonite Clay can be added to just about any recipe. We encourage you to experiment and try adding clay to all your favorite dishes. And when you create something great, please send us the recipe! We'll share it with all who are interested! You can email your recipes to Info@LivingClayBook.com.

Here are a few Calcium Bentonite Clay recipes to get you started. Bon Apetit!

Banana Nut Muffins
Ingredients:
1¼ cup flour
¼ cup dry powder Calcium Bentonite Clay
1½ tsp baking powder
¼ tsp baking soda
1/3 tsp salt
2 egg whites
1 cup mashed bananas
3/4 cup sugar
1 Tbs vegetable oil
1 tsp lemon zest
¼ cup chopped walnuts

Preheat oven to 350° F. Spray muffin tins with non-stick cooking spray. Stir together flour, Calcium Bentonite Clay, baking powder, soda and salt. In a medium bowl, beat egg whites slightly. Stir in bananas, sugar, oil, and lemon peel. Add to flour mixture and stir until just combines. Stir in walnuts. Fill muffin tins ¾ full. Bake for 20-25 minutes.

Banana Peanut Butter Chocolate Shake

Ingredients:

1 frozen banana, peeled

3 Tablespoons chocolate syrup (I use sugar-free)

1 cup milk

1 Tablespoon peanut butter

1 Tablespoon Dry Powder Calcium Bentonite Clay

2 ice cubes

Blend all ingredients until very smooth. Pour into a chilled glass and enjoy!

Beef Stew

Ingredients:

2 tablespoons all-purpose flour

1 pound beef or pork stew meat, cut into 3/4-inch cubes

2 tablespoons cooking oil

1/2 cup Liquid Calcium Bentonite Clay

2 1/2 cups cubed potatoes

1 cup frozen cut green beans

1 cup frozen whole kernel corn

1 cup sliced carrot

1 medium onion, cut into thin wedges

2 teaspoons instant beef bouillon granules

2 teaspoons Worcestershire sauce

1 teaspoon dried oregano, crushed

1/2 teaspoon dried marjoram or basil, crushed

1/4 teaspoon pepper

1 bay leaf

2 1/2 cups vegetable juice or hot-style vegetable juice

Directions

1. Place flour in a plastic bag. Add meat cubes and shake until meat is coated with flour. In a large skillet brown half of the meat in 1 tablespoon of the hot oil, turning to brown evenly. Brown remaining meat in remaining oil. Drain off fat.

2. In a 3 1/2 or 4 quart crockery cooker layer potatoes, green beans, corn, carrot, and onion. Add meat. Add bouillon granules, Worcestershire sauce, oregano, marjoram, pepper, and bay leaf. Pour vegetable juice and liquid Calcium Bentonite Clay over all.

3. Cover and cook on low-heat setting for 10 to 12 hours or on high-heat setting for 5 to 6 hours or until meat and vegetables are tender. Discard bay leaf. Ladle into bowls. Makes 4 to 6 servings.

Berry Muffins
   Ingredients:
   ¾ cup whole wheat flour
   1 cup all purpose flour
   ¼ cup Dry Powder Calcium Bentonite Clay
   1/3 cup wheat germ
   2/3 cup white sugar
   1 Tbs baking powder
   1 tsp salt
   1 tsp cinnamon
   2 eggs, beaten
   2 cups half & half cream
   1 cup fresh blackberries
   1 cup fresh blueberries
Preheat oven to 400° F. Butter muffin pan. Whisk together flour, Calcium Bentonite Clay, wheat germ, sugar, baking powder, salt and cinnamon. In another bowl whisk together half & half cream and eggs. Stir wet ingredients into dry ingredients, mixing just to combine. Fold in berries. Scoop batter into muffin pan cups 2/3 full. Bake in preheated oven for 20 minutes or until done.

TLC Breakfast Elixir
   This is like a super-souped-up smoothie. A great way to ENERGIZE your day!

Soaked almonds – 8-10
4-5 small pieces of fresh chunk coconut
Generous sprinkling of flax seed
a few chopped Brazil nuts
Blend these with 4-8 ozs water
Next add: (Pick from different ones for variety but use lots
of greens.)
Orange or grapefruit - leave pith on
Apples
Pineapple
Banana or 1 plantain
Seasonal fruits
Tamarind – 1" cube
Seeded grapes - a few
Celery chopped
Bean sprouts - handful
Snow peas - a few chopped

Lettuce - kale, chard, spinach leaf, endive red tip lettuce
Cucumber
Liquid Calcium Bentonite Clay 2 oz.
Blend together until smooth. ENJOY!

Brownies
Ingredients:
1 ½ cups unsalted butter
3 cups white sugar
2 tsp vanilla
7 eggs
1 cup flour
¼ cup Dry Powder Calcium Bentonite Clay
1 ¼ cups unsweetened cocoa powder
1 tsp salt
1 cup chopped walnuts
Preheat oven to 350° F. Line a 9x9 pan with foil and spray
with cooking spray. In a saucepan over medium heat, melt but-

ter. Stir in sugar until dissolved. Remove mixture from heat and beat in the eggs one at a time mixing well after each addition. Stir in vanilla. Sift dry ingredients together. Add the flour mixture to the butter mixture and mix until combined. Stir in walnuts and spread batter into the pan. Bake at 350° F for 45-50 minutes. Do not over bake.

Guacamole

Ingredients:
2 Ripe Avocados
1 tablespoon Hydrated Calcium Bentonite Clay
1 Clove garlic — Mashed
3 tablespoons lime juice
1 jalapeno — Seeded, Diced
2 Tomatoes — seeded and chopped
1 Small Red Onion — chopped fine
1/4 cup cilantro leaves — finely chopped
Salt and freshly ground pepper

153

Halve and pit avocados and scoop flesh into a large bowl. Mash avocado with a fork and mix in the hydrated Calcium Bentonite Clay. Stir in remaining ingredients, combining well. Chill covered with plastic wrap for at least 1 hour and up to 1 day. Stir guacamole well and serve with tortilla chips.

Honey Water

2 cups of water
1 healing teaspoon of Powder Calcium Bentonite Clay
4 tsp raw honey
Put in a plastic or glass container with a plastic lid. Shake well and drink.

Lemon Meringue Pie

Ingredients:
1 (9 inch) pie crust, baked
1 1/2 cups white sugar

1/2 teaspoon salt
1 1/2 cups water
1/2 cup cornstarch
1/4 cup Dry Powder Calcium Bentonite Clay
1/3 cup water
4 eggs, separated
1/2 cup lemon juice
2 teaspoons lemon zest
3 tablespoons butter
1/4 teaspoon salt
1/2 cup white sugar
Preheat oven to 325 degrees F (165 degrees C).

Combine 1 1/2 cups sugar, salt, and 1 1/2 cups water in a heavy saucepan. Place over high heat and bring to a boil. In a small bowl, mix cornstarch, Calcium Bentonite Clay and 1/3 cup water to make a smooth paste. Gradually whisk into boiling sugar mixture. Boil mixture until thick and clear, stirring

constantly. Remove from heat. In a small bowl, whisk together egg yolks and lemon juice. Gradually whisk egg yolk mixture into hot sugar mixture. Return pan to heat and bring to a boil, stirring constantly. Remove from heat and stir in grated lemon rind and butter or margarine. Place mixture in refrigerator and cool until just lukewarm. In a large glass or metal bowl, combine egg whites and salt. Whip until foamy. Gradually add 1/2 cup sugar while continuing to whip. Beat until whites form stiff peaks. Stir about 3/4 cup of meringue into lukewarm filling. Spoon filling into baked pastry shell. Cover pie with remaining meringue. Bake in preheated oven for 15 minutes, until meringue is slightly brown. Cool on a rack at for at least 1 hour before cutting.

Mud Cake
Ingredients:
3/4 cup flour
1/4 cup Dry Powder Calcium Bentonite Clay

2 Tbs. cocoa
2 tsp. baking powder
½ tsp salt
½ cup milk
2 Tbs. salad oil
1 tsp. vanilla
¾ cup chopped pecans
Sauce:
¾ cup brown sugar
¼ cup cocoa
1 ¾ cup hot water

Mix the first five ingredients. Add milk, oil and vanilla and stir and mix well. Mix in nuts. Pour into a greased 8" Pyrex pan. Mix sauce and pour over the batter. Bake at 350° degree F for 35-40 minutes.

Oatmeal Cookies

Ingredients:

1 cup shortening
1 cup sugar
1 cup brown sugar
½ cup Dry Powder Calcium Bentonite Clay
2 eggs, beaten
1 tsp. vanilla
1 tsp. soda
1 cup flour
3 cups 3-Minute Oatmeal

Cream shortening, adding sugar gradually and mixing well. Mix soda, flour and Calcium Bentonite Clay and add to creamed mixture. Next add oats. Form into small balls and bake at 375° F. for 10-15 minutes. Makes 5 doz.

Pecan Sticks

1/8 cup butter
4 Tbs sugar

1 Tbs water
2 tsp. vanilla
½ cup Dry Powder Calcium Bentonite Clay
1 ½ cups. flour
1 cup pecans – chopped

Cream butter and sugar. Add flour and Calcium Bentonite Clay. Mix and blend together. Add water and vanilla. Add pecans. Press into a buttered 9x9 pan and bake at 325° F 10-12 minutes or until done. Cool and slice into sticks.

Refried Bean Dip

Ingredients:
1 lg. can refried beans
1 jar picante or taco sauce
1/4 Cup Hydrated Calcium Bentonite Clay
Sour cream
Chopped red peppers
Olives (black)
Shredded cheese
Fritos or Tortilla Chips

Mix refried beans with picante sauce and Calcium Bentonite Clay. Spread on serving tray. Cover with sour cream and shredded cheese. Add chopped red peppers and sliced black olives. Serve with chips. Serves 8 to 12.

Sugar Cookies

Ingredients:
1 cup sugar
½ cup Dry Powder Calcium Bentonite Clay
2 ½ cups flour
1 ½ tsp baking powder
1 cup shortening
3 Tbs. cream
1 tsp. vanilla

Blend dry ingredients together and add shortening. Mix together and add cream and vanilla. Dough may be chilled. Roll in a ball and mash with the bottom of a glass. Sprinkle lightly with sugar. Bake at 400° F for about 5-6 minutes.

Super Easy Cookies
Ingredients:
1 roll Pillsbury's Cookie Dough, any flavor
1/4 cup Dry Powder Calcium Bentonite Clay
Directions:
Unwrap cookie dough and set it in a bowl at room temperature to soften. Once softened, mix in the Calcium Bentonite Clay. Place by tablespoons on a cookie sheet, and bake as directed on the package. Couldn't be easier!

Wheat Pizza Dough
Ingredients:
1 tsp sugar
1½ cups warm water
1 Tbs active dry yeast
1 Tbs olive oil
1 tsp salt
2 cups whole-wheat flour
½ cup Dry Powder Calcium Bentonite Clay
1 cup flour

Dissolve sugar in water, sprinkle yeast over the top and let stand for about 10 minutes until foamy. Stir in olive oil and salt. Mix whole-wheat flour, Calcium Bentonite Clay and all-purpose flour until dough starts to come together. Knead dough on a well-floured surface. This takes about 10 minutes. Place dough in oiled bowl, cover with a towel and let rise for about an hour. When dough is doubled, put dough back on floured surface and divide into pieces for 2 thin crust or leave whole for thick crust. Form into a tight ball. Let it rise again for 45 minutes. Preheat oven to 425° F. Roll dough into desired

pizza shape. Place on a well-oiled surface, top pizza with favorite toppings and sauce. Bake for 16-20 minutes until crust
is golden.

LIVING CLAY AND AGELESS BEAUTY
How to look and feel 29 for 100+ years!

Longevity and beauty...No two attributes are more greatly coveted than these in our society. More money is spent, more experts consulted, and more energy expended on this elusive quest than any other.

I would contend that there is probably no one among those reading this book that is completely satisfied with both the way their body is aging (the speed, the look, the feel) and with their perceived appearance, their beauty...I want to suggest to you that you can actually reverse the aging process and change your appearance dramatically if you adopt the practices outlined in this chapter.

I believe everyone should live to be a minimum of 150-200 years old – in this very day and age – and should look and feel 29 until their 100th birthday.

We will look at what makes our bodies age. We will discuss the difference between positive and negative ionic charged molecules and how they relate to the aging process. We will define the "dying process" and the "living process." And finally we will outline the simple life plan that will add many, many years to your life – all the while, remaining one of the "pretty people."

Let's begin by taking a fun look at our beliefs about health. I can think of no better reflection of those beliefs than how we personally treat our own diseases and ailments. And what better evidence of that than to take...

...A PEEK IN YOUR MEDICINE CABINET!

Okay, be honest with me for a minute...really brutally honest...If I were to slip into your bathroom unnoticed and take a peek in your medicine cabinet – what would it say about your state of health, and even more importantly, what would it say about your core beliefs about health itself?

Let's take a look and see for ourselves...Go ahead, don't be shy...or embarrassed...everyone's looks about the same...

Reach up to that mirror and swing it open! That's it...Let's start with the top shelf...

There's Anacin, Excedrin, Excedrin P.M., Contac, Gelusil, Tylenol and a large old blue jar of Vicks. Then there's a bottle of Vivarin, a bottle of Serutan (that's Natures spelled backwards) and 2 bottles of Milk of Magnesia – the regular that tastes like liquid chalk and the mint flavor which tastes like mint-flavored liquid chalk. And here's a large bottle of Rolaids standing close to its friend, a large bottle of Tums. And the Tums are standing next to a large bottle of orange-flavored Di-Gel tablets. What a trio of acid-indigestion piggy banks they make...

Oh my, look at that second shelf and all of those vitamins! You got your A, your C, and your C with rosehips. You got your B-simple and B-complex and B-12. There's L-Lysine, which was supposed to have done something about those embarrassing skin problems, but hasn't, and Lecithin, which was supposed to remove cholesterol from your heart, but didn't. There's iron, calcium, and cod-liver oil. There's One-A-Day multiples, Myadec multiples, Centrum multiples. And sitting on top of the cabinet is a gigantic bottle of Geritol, just for good measure.

On the third shelf we find the utility infielders of the OTC medicine world. Ex-lax, Carter's Little Pills – both to keep you moving the mail. Next, we find Kaopectate, Pepto-Bismol and Preparation H, in case the mail moves too fast or too painfully. And some Tucks in a screw-top jar to keep the mailroom tidy after delivery has been made. There's Formula 44 for coughs, Nyquil and Dristan for colds, and a big bottle of castor oil. There's a tin of Sucrets and a quartet of mouthwashes: Chloraseptic, Cepacol, Cipastal in the spray bottle, and of course

Listerine – old faithful herself. Visine and Murine for the eyes. Cortaid and Neosporin ointment for the skin. A tub of Oxy-5 and a plastic bottle of Oxy-Wash for a few less zits and some tetracycline pills. And standing as the sentry in the back corner to the right is a bottle of coal-tar shampoo.

That narrow bottom shelf is known as the "serious business" shelf and is almost deserted. There's Valium, Percodan, Elavil and Darvon Complex. There's Ritalin, oh that magical gift from the Gods. There's a toothbrush in a travel tube and a tube of Crest Super White toothpaste. And then there's another Sucrets box on this low shelf, but there are no Sucrets in it. If you were to open it you would find six, year old Quaaludes – this is the emergency arsenal that will cure what ails you – at least till the sun rises...

Well now, quite a picture of balanced health, aren't we? Only one question remains—is there anything that can't be replaced with a daily regimen of Calcium Bentonite Clay? Go ahead, take a close look and see what you think. What would life be like with a medicine cabinet, which contained only primary curatives: Dry Powder Calcium Bentonite Clay, Hydrated Calcium Bentonite Clay Creamy Paste, and Liquid Calcium Bentonite Clay?

No, no, don't worry, I'm only joking of course...You couldn't really throw out everything in your medicine cabinet and replace it with Calcium Bentonite Clay...or could you?

As you ponder the remoteness of that even being a possibility, let's shift gears and look at our bodies on a cellular level. What is it that causes each and every little-bitty cell to live or die at any given moment?

Science has shown that the effects of detoxification on our body's cells are nothing short of miraculous. The following is an excerpt from Natasha Lee's article "Could Detoxification be the Fountain of Youth?"

"Dr. Alexis Carrel, of the Rockefeller Institute for Medical Research performed an amazing experiment in the early

1900's. He managed to sustain the life of cells from a chicken embryo by immersing them in a solution containing all the nutrients necessary for life and changed the solution daily. The cells took up nutrients from the nutrient-rich broth and excreted their wastes into the same solution. The only thing Dr. Carrel did each day was discard the old solution and replace it with fresh nutrient solution. The chicken cells lived for 29 years until one night Dr. Carrel's assistant forgot to change the polluted solution! We do not know how much longer the cell's life could have been maintained.

Dr Carrel concluded at the end of his experiment that the cell is actually immortal. It is merely the fluid in which it floats which degenerates. He is quoted saying, "The cell is immortal, renew this fluid at intervals, give the cell something on which to feed and, so far as we know, the pulsation of life may go on forever." The average chicken lives about 7 years. His detoxified, properly nourished chicken cell lived for 29 years.

It may be hard to believe that the body could live indefinitely, however, a similar level of vibrant health and life extension can be created in humans by following the obvious similar principal.

Every cell in our body excretes waste material that becomes toxic, and poisonous to our bodies if we allow it to build up faster than we renew the fluid in which it floats. According to the above experiment, this is the cause of aging and degeneration. Factors such as "time" and ideas such as as "that's just life" fade from the picture, with new data in view. The fact is, every 7 years we have a completely new set of bones, teeth, skin and hair. Logically, a person should be able to look and feel better than they did 7 years ago by changing and improving the way they take care of their own body as Dr. Carrel took care of his chicken cell.

Time alone is not a disease or poison, it is the toxins that accumulate with time that the body cannot withstand that in turn causes deterioration. In other words, time alone is not the cause of death. Poisons are the cause of death of life forms.

So logically, and from the above data by detoxifying your cells, a person can freshen up and grow healthier and younger than they once were by practicing this principle. Periodically detoxifying the body, drinking lots of fresh water and staying smart on nutrition can appear to work miracles. Dr. Carrel however proved these amazing results are not miracles, just good science."

So if time alone does not cause the death of us at a cellular level, and assuming that poisons, toxins, and the like do – what if…just what if, we could consistently and completely rid our bodies of all poisons, toxins and any other environmental malady of our own creation, on a consistent basis? Just what if…

AMINO ACIDS – ANOTHER KEY TO AGELESSNESS

Amino acids are the building blocks of life that make up proteins, which are essential to life. They are a primary ingredient of most cell structures. Proteins are essential to all the chemical processes of the cells and thus are needed to rebuild the constant wear and tear on the human body. For instance, high-protein diets are especially vital during the growth years, during pregnancy, and when tissue has been damaged by injury or disease.

Some research has shown that Calcium Bentonite Clay may have played an essential role in the formation of life. This hypothesis comes from experiments performed with clay to recreate the conditions under which amino acids may form proteins. In the laboratory, tests showed that single amino acids formed into the longer chains called peptides on the surface of clay particles. The clay is thought to act as a pattern and catalyst for the formation of long peptide chains, or proteins. Scientists added a small amount of one amino acid to a solution of various clay minerals. They then exposed the clay to varying degrees of temperature and moisture. The main findings were that more peptides were produced at various temperatures when clay was present than when it was absent. And that the production of peptides was higher in the presence of the changes in temperature and moisture. Protein conversion can sometimes fail to proceed normally through the peptide chains in the human body and, as a result, prevent their use.

On the basis of these finding, published in *Scientific American* (Millot 1979), the investigators proposed that the fluctuation of temperature and moisture brings about a distribution and redistribution of amino acids on the surface of clay particles that favors the amino acids' linkage into peptide chains. When moisture touches the surface of the clay mineral, the active sites on the surface that speed the formulation of peptides are cleaned. Then, when the same water used to clean the surface evaporates because of the change in temperature, new catalytic sites become available for other amino acids to form new chains. This ongoing cycle, totally dependent upon the clay minerals, is synonymous with life.

The summation is an easy one: Clay is synonymous with life. Clay produces more peptides, and in turn, more protein amino acid links to life forming peptide chains.

THE IMPORTANCE OF pH

The pH of Calcium Bentonite Clay can be as high as 9.7, and thus it acts as an alkalizing agent in the body. The pH scales goes from 0 to 14, with 7 being neutral. Below 7 is acid and above 7 is alkaline. The body's pH level plays a critical role in its ability to remain healthy and resist disease. Tissues in the body that are poorly oxygenated, or devoid of oxygen, are acidic and prone to disease. Cancerous tissues are acidic, whereas healthy tissues are alkaline. Blood, lymph and cerebral spinal fluid in the human body are designed to be slightly alkaline at a pH of 7.4. At a pH level of 7.4 cancer cells become dormant and at a pH 8.5 cancer cells will die while healthy cells will live. Disease occurs when pH falls into the acid range. It is essential to alkalize the body, to a pH of 7.4 or slightly above, by every means available.

To recap: Cancer cells become dormant at a pH of 7.4 and die at a pH of 8.5! Look for Calcium Bentonite Clays that have a pH range of 9.5 or higher. Calcium Bentonite Clay effectively raises the pH of your body to whatever level you choose based on how it is used.

ARE WE FIGHTING THE WRONG WAR?

We view the problem of illness as something we should attack, something we should declare war on...The metaphor of declaring "war on..." is not limited to medicine. In recent years, we have declared a war on crime, a war on drugs, a war on AIDS, and so on. I do not believe that looking at disease from this perspective has been any more successful than any of the other "wars on" we have declared. In fact, I believe a declaration of war insures the problem will stay with us in perpetuity.

Our current health policy, dictated by the giant pharmaceutical companies, waits for a disease to occur and then attempts to kill and poison it out of our bodies in a full frontal attack. Perhaps we are now realizing, after almost a 100 year failed experiment, this approach may not have proven itself to be in our best interest. Is it today time to resort to a more intelligent medical treatment system? Is it time to shift the emphasis to health preservation and longevity, rather than treatment of disease after the fact and acceptance of death at 78.5 years of age – the last five years of that having fought the "war on" heart disease or the "war on" cancer?

CLAY IS ALIVE!

Raymond Dextreit, the French naturopath who popularized clay curative in his country, says the following: "One of clay's peculiarities is based on its physical-chemical domination. From a thermodynamic point of view, we must admit that clay cannot be the sole source of energy of the phenomena it produces. Clay is effective as a dynamic presence far more significantly than a mere consideration of the substances it contains. It is a catalyst rather than an agent itself. This is possible because clay is alive."

THE ENERGY OF CLAY!

If we go back to our base physical components, we can safely say that we are built from multitudes of particles held together by electrical bonds. Electrical forces are what hold atoms and molecules together. Chemical bonds and reactions depend on these electrical forces. Therefore, all chemical reactions are, in essence, reorganizations of electrical forces, which continue to be vital at body levels, i.e., tissues and organs. When this is all taken into account, a living organism is shown to be an extremely intricate electrical system (Gibson and Gibson 1987).

During illness, the vital force is weak and incapable of supporting the body and its functions. In health, however, the opposite occurs: the force is strong and is able to counteract sickness and decay. What keeps the immune system running is the energy that feeds it, the substance of life. The body will not run well, or will at least run with all sorts of mechanical problems, when there is no energy to support it.

When clay is consumed, its vital force is released into the physical body and mingles with the vital energy of the body, creating a stronger, more powerful energy in the host. Its particles are catalysts for stimulation and transformation capable of withholding and releasing energy at impulse. The natural magnetic action transmits a remarkable power to the organism and helps to rebuild vital potential through the liberation of latent energy. When it is in contact with the body, its very nature compels it to release its vital force: the same vital force from which so many plants and animals feed.

Therefore, in order to create health, the body must be stimulated and restimulated by another working energy like clay. When the immune system does not function at its best, the clay stimulates the body's inner resources to awaken the stagnant energy. It supplies the body with the available magnetism to run well.

Clay is said to propel the immune system to find a new healthy balance. Reactions are not forced, but rather triggered into effect, as they are needed. To put it into other words, clay simply strengthens the body to a point of higher resistance. In this way, the body's natural immune system has an improved chance of restoring and maintaining health.

According to Dr. Robert T. Martin, PhD, Cornell University, and Mineralogist, MIT, one gram of Calcium Bentonite Clay has a surface area of over 800 square meters. The greater the surface area, the greater the adsorption and in turn the greater its power to attract positively charged particles/molecules.

Dr. Martin further reports in the same study that Calcium Bentonite Clay gives no evidence that it has any chemical effect on the body. Its action is purely physical. Due to its huge surface area and negative charge, it maintains its molecular whole and does not break down or assimilate with the body.

He commented at a recent conference, "One marvels at what Calcium Bentonite Clay can do. For something that is merely an inert matter, it gives quite a performance. The same teaspoon of clay can cure an obstinate carbuncle and tenacious anemia equally well. Curing the carbuncle is easily explained by clay's absorbent power…but anemia – that's part of the magic of Living Clay…it simply transforms living energetic matter!"

We must accept the facts even if we do not understand their origin. And clay does act with wisdom – it goes to the unhealthy spot. Used internally, whether absorbed orally, anally or vaginally, clay goes to the place where harm is, there it lodges, perhaps for several days, until finally it draws out the toxins, disease, etc., with its evacuation.

From helping to prevent the proliferation of pathogenic germs and parasites to aiding with rebuilding of healthy tissues and cells, clay is a 'living' cure.

And finally, from Dr. Robert Whittaker, M.D., Cornell University, "Calcium Bentonite Clay transmits a remarkable life energy to the organism, helping to rebuild vital potential through the liberation of latent energy. When the immune system is under attack and not functioning at its best, Calcium Bentonite Clay stimulates the body's inner resources to awaken the stagnant energy. It supplies the body with the necessary negative ionic charge to run well. Calcium Bentonite Clay propels the immune system to a healthy balance and strengthens the body to its point of highest resistance. Calcium Bentonite Clay restores and rejuvenates the body on a cellular energetic level, essentially reversing the traditional dying process to one of a living rejuvenation process. Calcium Bentonite Clay literally turns the dying and aging process upside down and turns back the hands of time in life's time continuum.

We have answered a few of the questions presented early on in this chapter regarding longevity. I now want to shift gears a bit and discuss the "ageless beauty" aspect of Calcium Bentonite Clay.

While beauty is only skin deep, the effects of Calcium Bentonite Clay touch your body on every level. As one young Calcium Bentonite Clay user told me, "It's helped me from head to toe, from stem to stern, and from all the way inside to all the way out." I don't think I could have said it better myself!

One of my great joys in life has been in watching first hand the dramatic effect Calcium Bentonite Clay has had on the complexion of young teens. The transformation in these lives is a sight to behold. There have been times when the change in complexion and look is so dramatic I failed to recognize the client. One of those clients whom I met several years ago during a Los Angeles area event stands out for me. It was my first eyewitness account of such a transformation.

A young girl of maybe 13 or 14 years, was standing with her mother, head bowed, bangs covering her forehead, looking at the Calcium Bentonite Clay and the specialty beauty products of a Calcium Bentonite Clay company. She could be described as a plain looking girl with pretty eyes. After a few minutes of shuffling back and forth and asking her mother to get her some Calcium Bentonite Clay, the mother looked to me and said, "Hey, do you think the clay will help her?" The mother put her hand under her daughter's chin and although met with some resistance, the daughter's face was slowly raised to the light. The embarrassed daughter's eyes closed as her severe case of acne soon became apparent to all...

To make a two month story much shorter I found myself once again in L.A. at a similar event, and after speaking went to the back of the room to answer questions privately. A young girl came running up and gave me a big hug. She looked up into my eyes and said it worked! It really worked! I was struggling to remember who she might be and just what it was that had worked. At that same moment, I caught with the corner of my eyes someone walking up whom I did recognize...It was the mother of the young girl I met 2 months prior with the severe case of acne. I looked back to the girl and realized that in fact it really had worked – oh yes, it really, really had worked...

Standing before me was a completely transformed young lady. Her hair was pulled back off her forehead, eyes wide open and sparkling and a bright beaming smile like I had never before seen met mine. AND absolutely the most perfect, smooth, radiant complexion you had ever laid eyes on...not a trace of acne remained...

In that moment when she knew that I knew who she was, the story began gushing out. In a few seconds her mother arrived and she too began her version of the transformation. With both of them simulcasting their own version of the story, I don't believe I understood anything further that was said by either. What I can still hear clearly today are the words that really mattered…"It worked! It really worked!"

That story in many similar versions has played out in my life countless times over the past few years; the transformations just as dramatic in each individual life, just different cities, and different names.

Today, spas and resorts around the world are touting Calcium Bentonite Clay as a true miracle. One Medi-Spa in California calls their Calcium Bentonite Clay facial treatments "Botox in a jar." The results are truly astounding. Based on Calcium Bentonite Clay's huge success in the Spa and Beauty industry, one innovative Calcium Bentonite Clay company created an entire cosmeceutical line of body creams, lotions and anti-aging products. All have as a base ingredient their pure, all natural Calcium Bentonite Clay. This is truly a unique line of products and one of the fastest selling new lines in the Spa/Resort/Beauty industry.

The good news is that you have a choice. You can choose to experience the age-reversing effects of Calcium Bentonite Clay at Spas and Resorts across the United States, or you can purchase Calcium Bentonite Clay online and enjoy all its benefits for only pennies on the dollar in the privacy of your own home. A full and complete line of Calcium Bentonite Clay based beauty treatment products is now available to everyone.

Clinics and Medi-Spas are literally taking 10, 20, even 30 years off their clients in as little as 3-4 complete treatments. A comment from a client who had received 4 weekly Calcium Bentonite Clay treatments and who had as well completed a 30 day full body detox and internal cleanse said, "Look at me!… In the past 30 days I have taken 20 years off of the way I look and feel. My complexion is absolutely radiant – all of my wrinkles are gone! My body is firm and tighter, my energy level up. I'm 52 years old and look and feel 29 again…Many of my friends aren't even recognizing me anymore. This is an absolute miracle in my life…"

Is it only a coincidence that the most recent reports of people living to be 150+ years old come from an Indian tribe who's elders lived in Calcium Bentonite Clay caves?

What if you could actually live in your own clay house? Ever since I first visited the ancient Indian Clay Cave houses near Shoshone, California, I've wanted to find a way to incorporate Living Clay into modern day home building. I considered cutting stone blocks or tile slabs but the mineral is too soft for construction purposes and would wear much too easily unless used as a finish or decorative touch of sorts…Then one day the light came on and today a new product is available which will allow you to literally build and finish out your home with clay. You can build your very own healthy "green" negative ionic charged house – or remodel the one you now own.

The latest and hottest new wall treatment on the market is a unique clay product that's all about adding a beautiful earth texture, with a touch of color, while creating a healthier environment for you and your family. It's a new Living Clay plaster that can easily mimic the rugged earthy feel of adobe or the smooth porcelain finish of Venetian plaster. It takes the place of traditional plaster, but has the added benefit of being easier to install and repair. It is breathable, flexible, mold-resistant, and dust free – and it can be used on walls or ceilings.

It's also backed by an eco-friendly philosophy. People are drawn to this clay because it is "green." It's a formulation of natural Living Clay, Zeolite clay, and recycled aggregates and was developed specifically to take the place of traditional plaster. Not only is Living Clay environmentally friendly, it sets up a unique environment in the home. It invokes a calm, soothing environment. If the clay is left unsealed, you're setting up a really different environment in the room. Most building products used in home construction produce positive ions, so there is constantly a charge in our environment. Living Clay produces negative ions. The balance actually aids in controlling the climate of a room. The clay naturally regulates arid and humid air by absorbing and releasing moisture as conditions change.

There has been a huge response for this new product. Homeowners have been hungry for something like this – easy to use, "green," and gives them the warmth and even more versatility than plaster.

It's very user friendly and can be applied by novices as well as professional plasterers because it's so much easier than traditional plaster. It can be used on any room in the house, but is not recommended for specific areas that come in direct contact with water. With the proper sealer it can be used in areas that receive some direct moisture. It works well over existing plasters, drywall, brick and concrete and covers a multitude of sins in older homes.

It can pretty much go over any surface as long as it's primed properly with a sanded primer. Do-it-yourselfers simply mix the powder clay with water, add any desired tint and trowel it onto their walls or ceiling. It really is that easy – and if you make a mistake you can fix it even days later. It's very forgiving. You can rework it days after to get the finish you want. You can actually rewet it and rework it.

Once homeowners are satisfied with its looks, the plaster can be sealed or left as is. Once you seal it you can clean it with a damp sponge, but I like to keep it as natural as possible. To me, that is really the essence of the Living Clay product.

The entire process is rather quick. A homeowner can easily refinish a single, average size room in a weekend. It's a very user-friendly product. It makes people feel like they're doing something that is aesthetically beautiful while at the same time environmentally friendly for their home and family. The day has come that you can now live in your very own Living Clay home and experience the ageless beautify and ageless benefits of its magical gifts.

Is it only a coincidence that the only other historical find of the same type of 100% pure Calcium Bentonite Clay was made on the west and south sides of the Dead Sea, where hundreds of Biblical accounts recorded people living to be 600 to 900 years old?

This book is jam-packed full of scientific evidence and real life testimonies attesting to the miracle of Calcium Bentonite Clay. I could go on and on for pages playing the "Is it only a coincidence" game. All evidence clearly points to one thing – that ageless beauty and longevity are no coincidence when Calcium Bentonite Clay is used as a life practice – it is a truth!

Choose to live to be 150+ years old! Choose to feel 29 while doing so! Choose to take responsibility for your health and lifestyle choices! Choose Calcium Bentonite Clay!

Now go play in your clay!

RESOURCE LISTING

This book is intended as a resource to inform the reader of many of the various uses for Calcium Bentonite Clay. It is not intended as a sales or marketing tool, or for product endorsement. FDA and FTC regulations prohibit this type of endorsement when discussing curative or treatment methods.

What the below reference listing is intended to do is to refer you to several sources of information which may assist you in your search for the best Calcium Bentonite Clay available today.

Our first suggestion is to do a "Google Search" (or Yahoo or any other leading search engine) using the search parameters of "Calcium Bentonite Clay." The results of this search should give you several sources, which I would recommend you either email or phone with any questions you may have. And remember to ask the questions outlined in the book to insure that you are getting the best available product. In a recent search for "Calcium Bentonite Clay," I learned there were over 34,000 hits for those search parameters. I also learned that the top companies, in my opinion, came up in the top 5-6 listings in this search as well.

In addition to a Google Search, we also want to refer you to three excellent independent resources for further information on Calcium Bentonite Clay. These sites offer a wealth of information and possibly offer you further suggestions as to what and where to buy the best available Living Clay. They are as follows:

www.AboutClay.com
www.EytonsEarth.org
www.shirleys-wellness-cafe.com

Above all else, I encourage you to take responsibility for your own health. Don't allow another day to pass without Clay in it. I promise you will experience a better quality of life as soon as you make the choice to use clay on a daily basis, and you just may live to be 100+ and still look 29.

Now, go drink some clay.

178

Living Clay Order Form

Item	Price	Quantity	Total
Living Clay – Nature's Own Miracle Cure Book	20.00		

Please send Check, Money Order or Credit Card Authorization to: Accepting MasterCard, Visa and Discover **Perry A~** 626 Scheel Kyle, TX 78640 1-866-883-1591 PH: 512.262-7187 FX: 512.532.6086 Email: PerryA@Austin.rr.com www.LivingClayBook.com	Sub-Total For Order	$
	Texas Tax @ 8.25%	$
	US Priority mail (up to 3 items) w/ Delivery Conformation	$ 4.60
	Additional items @ $1.00 each	
	TOTAL	$

Mail to Name: _____   Phone: (____) _____

Address: _____

City: _____   State: _____   Zip: _____

182

Email for Conformation Number: _____
(For Credit Card Orders)
Name as it appears on card: _____

Signature: _____

Credit card Type: Visa _____   Mastercard _____   American Express _____

Card Number: _____   Expiration date:_____

Please autograph as follows:_____

Thank You!